Prevention is the keyword in Dr. Francisco Contreras's fight against disease. This book will provide the steps to you to strengthen your heart and prevent cardiovascular disease. I fully recommend that you read this book, but more importantly, I encourage you to apply its principles to your daily life.

−Dr. Mario Zuniga
Cardiologist

Francisco Contreras, M.D., is the most knowledgeable and compassionate doctor I know. He and his medical staff at the Oasis of Hope Hospital have helped me with my heart health tremendously.

−Dr. Richard Shakarian
International President
Full Gospel Business Men's Fellowship International

Francisco Contreras, M.D., has helped me achieve health goals when other doctors were unable to. His ability to combine medicine, nutrition and spirituality sets him apart from everyone in his field.

−Denice Shakarian Halicki
Executive Producer
Gone In 60 Seconds (Touchstone Pictures)

This book is also very useful for people who have had heart problems in whatever stage they may be in.

−Dr. Lorenzo A. Arce-Piña
Cardiologist
Professor of Cardiology

Individuals must assume responsibility for their own health. In this book, Dr. Contreras proposes lifestyle changes that will benefit your cardiovascular condition.

−Dr. Juan José Parcero-Valdés
Cardiologist

A Healthy Heart

Francisco Contreras, M.D.

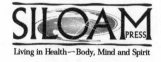

SILOAM PRESS

Living in Health—Body, Mind and Spirit

A Healthy Heart by Francisco Contreras, M.D.
Published by Siloam Press
A part of Strang Communications Company
600 Rinehart Road
Lake Mary, Florida 32746
www.siloampress.com

Unless otherwise noted, all Scripture quotations are from the Holy Bible, New King James Version. Copyright © 1979, 1980, 1982 by Thomas Nelson, Inc., publishers. Used by permission.

Scripture quotations marked KJV are from the King James Version of the Bible.

Scripture quotations marked NAS are from the New American Standard Bible. Copyright © 1960, 1962, 1963, 1968, 1971, 1972, 1973, 1975, 1977 by the Lockman Foundation. Used by permission. (www.Lockman.org)

Scripture quotations marked NIV are from the Holy Bible, New International Version. Copyright © 1973, 1978, 1984, International Bible Society. Used by permission.

Library of Congress Catalog Card Number: 2001090574
International Standard Book Number: 0-88419-765-4

This book is not intended to provide medical advice or to take the place of medical advice and treatment from your personal physician. Readers are advised to consult their own doctors or other qualified health professionals regarding the treatment of their medical problems. Neither the publisher nor the author takes any responsibility for any possible consequences from any treatment, action or application of medicine, supplement, herb or preparation to any person reading or following the information in this book. If readers are taking prescription medications, again, they should consult with their physicians and not take themselves off of medicines to start supplementation without the proper supervision of a physician.

01 02 03 04 05   8 7 6 5 4 3 2 1
Printed in the United States of America

To my wife, Rosy—
"Wild thing . . .
you make my heart sing . . ."

Acknowledgements

The millenarian wisdom of the Chinese reveals that "all is known because all of us know something."

I'm indebted to Jorge Barroso-Aranda, Ph.D., M.D., for his extensive and accurate research work on the latest findings about the heart, its ailments, treatments and the power of nutrients to reverse cardiovascular disease. This knowledge will empower you to prevent the leading cause of death in America.

I want to thank Joel Kilpatrick for his fine work as writer and for his patience as we labored through the process of revisions.

Without the talent of Peg de Alminana, all the scientific truths in this book would be completely inaccessible to the lay reader and would be nothing but a boring account of scientific data. As project manager and writer/editor of this book, she has conveyed my ideas as if she were able to read my mind.

Deborah Moss's intelligent eye has grasped inconsistencies and errors and has constructed an impeccable text.

Luisa Ruiz, my cousin but also an insightful copyeditor of texts in Spanish, has helped me with the corrections on the contents of the book.

María Antonia Bernal, my quiet but merry secretary, patiently spent long hours typing medical articles.

I would also like to thank Judith McKittrick for applying her creativity in the design of the cover and Karen Judge for her usual meticulous fine job in typesetting.

Spreading the good news about a healthy heart will be possible thanks to the goal-and-strategy-oriented mind of Larry Bregel and his marketing team.

So many people put their heart in this book; to all of them I express my deepest gratitude.

Contents

Section II
Become Heart Smart—Keys to Developing
or Reclaiming a Healthy Heart

Foreword

A few years ago, I had the privilege of observing Dr. Contreras work with a patient. The patient was a woman who had a tumor the size of a watermelon on the back of her knee. Her doctor recommended amputating the affected leg up through the pelvis as a safety measure. Dr. Contreras agreed with the doctor that surgery was the best option, but he considered the quality of life of the patient, calculated the risk of metastasis with a more conservative approach, informed the patient and together they decided to remove only the tumor and leave the leg intact. Dr. Contreras operated on the woman's leg for six hours, carefully cutting out the cancer without severing tendons, veins, arteries and nerves. Two days after the surgery, the woman walked out of the hospital with the assistance of a cane. Six months later, Dr. Contreras received a picture of the woman walking on the beach with her son. What mattered most to this woman was not the recommended treatment, because both doctors recommended surgery. It was how the surgery was performed that made a tremendous difference to the quality of life that the woman is experiencing today.

Dr. Francisco Contreras's passion is to end needless suffering and to help people live the highest quality of life possible. He represents neither the conventional nor the alternative school of thought. His love and mission is for people, and he has dedicated his medical career to empowering them to make informed decisions about their health.

Dr. Contreras was classically trained in surgery at the University of Vienna in Austria, but he was exposed to the use of nutrition and holistic methods in his father's medical practice. He encourages everyone to be proactive about preventing illness. His belief in the power of knowledge has inspired his extensive research, writing and lecturing. Much like religious reformers who shared the sacred Scripture with the masses, Dr. Contreras collects health and illness data, statistics and reports and puts them into a context that is comprehensible and applicable by everyday, nonmedical, people. He travels every year to ten or more countries in keeping with his commitment to keep his patients informed.

A Healthy Heart is a product of Dr. Francisco Contreras's years of research and commitment to helping people maintain or regain health. It is very easy to read and understand. Each year, heart disease claims more lives in the USA than any other illness, including cancer. The information in this book is vital to you and your loved ones. It is comprehensive, concise and accurate. Dr. Contreras articulately explains how you can transition yourself into a low-risk group.

Few medical doctors integrate emotional and spiritual therapies into their patients' treatment courses. Dr. Contreras not only acknowledges the mind, body and spirit connection in this book, but he embraces it and expresses how you can bring the three realms into a healthy balance to help prevent a heart incident or improve your recovery from illness. You will enjoy reading this book; it can change your life. In fact, it can save your life, if you take Dr. Contreras's message to heart.

—Dr. Daniel E. Kennedy
CEO
Bio-Tec Group

Section I
With Every
Beat of My Heart

Chapter 1

What Is
Heart Disease?

E ven though it was fleeting, the experience of seeing a heart's crown come to life before my eyes for the first time was exhilarating. As a surgeon I had become familiar with the awesome marvel of a beating heart, even to hold it in my hands, but on March 15, 1985 I set foot for the first time into a "cath lab" (catheterization laboratory), an imposing room revealing man's incredible capacity to invent the most sophisticated of technologies. The heart of this room is an imposing C-shaped iron arm containing a fluoroscopic devise that allows real-time viewing of the heart's irrigation system.

By the time I walked in, my patient was already prepped and covered with sterile draping except for a small opening in the upper right thigh, which had been sterilized with an iodine solution to kill any bacteria and infiltrated with local anesthesia for the puncture that would introduce the catheter. The drapes were set as a tent at the patient's head level, and I could see his face. He smiled with a combination of relief and concern, happy that I was there with him at this time of trial. A catheter as thick as pencil lead was guided from the femoral artery in the groin all the way up into the "trunk," the origin, of the arteries that feed blood to the heart. Once the catheter was in place, the interventionist cardiologist instilled the contrast material allowing, albeit only for seconds, a web of vessels to reveal itself like a veil with the embroidery heavier at the top, a veil fit to cover the head of a king. Now I saw clearly why it was named the "crown." The arteries that form this veil were dubbed the coronaries.

> More than 2,600 deaths occur in the U.S. each day from cardiovascular disease—one death every 33 seconds.

The patient lay as still as possible, but his face revealed the questions and tension he felt about what the outcome might show. *Would more tests be required? How damaged was his heart? Would the cardiologists recommend some kind of immediate intervention?*

As the cardiologist released the dye through the catheter, for a split second the coronary system came into view on the x-ray screen.

As I watched, I was taken aback by its beauty, its form and its economy of design. The cardiologist mapped the branches of the coronaries as I stood there dazzled by the pumping organ. The complete evaluation came after a "movie" of the procedure was reviewed in slow motion to make a definitive diagnosis.

In this case, the crown of the patient's heart was so obviously damaged by plaque that even a novice like myself could see it. The slow-motion review merely confirmed what was very plain in the live study.

This heart was severely damaged and needed repairing.

My fascination gave way to heaviness in my own heart. Yes, it was the first time I had seen a live, beating heart, and I was completely enthralled. But the patient under the sterile draping was no stranger. He was my father.

As the catheter was removed from his leg, all the professional technicians and doctors were polite and courteous, but I could not help feeling the coldness of the event. The technology was astounding, but it lent a chill to the room, crowding out the humanness of my father's experience with dry detachment.

Because everyone knew it was my father, the final diagnosis and treatment recommendations were postponed, although everyone knew that something needed to be done to give him a few more years. The question was, What?

THIS UNCONTROLLED KILLER

Technology has come a long way in diagnosing and treating heart disease. Doctors see the heart as a machine to be treated and cured in the same way an automobile or a computer is repaired. We have emerged from the dark ages through an amazing array of mind-boggling machines and methods that would have been inconceivable just a few decades ago.

Yet with all this at our disposal, we have not conquered the menacing giant of heart disease. Interventions such as the ones above can save lives, but they do not completely solve the problem. Today's procedures are little more than sophisticated plumbing jobs that bypass a blockage but leave the disease intact. This devastating fact is lost in all the glitter of modern cardiac technology.

Before 1900, heart disease was not nearly the threat it is today.[1] More people worked jobs that required manual labor, which exercised the heart. Diets were better than they are now, and people tended to die of other causes before heart problems got them. In 1900, the leading causes of death were:

1. Pneumonia (including influenza)
2. Tuberculosis
3. Diarrhea (including other intestinal problems)
4. Heart disease

In 1901, heart disease became the third greatest killer. In 1908, it was number two. In 1910, it became the number one cause of death in America, and it has remained so ever since, except during the flu epidemic of 1918–1920.[2]

Not only did the incidence of heart disease increase, but also it increased at an alarming rate. By 1959, heart disease claimed more lives than the next four causes of death combined, including cancer and automobile accidents.[3] The rate of heart disease increased so sharply between 1940 and 1967 that the World Health Organization called it the world's most serious epidemic.[4]

Even though atherosclerosis—hardening of the arteries—was well established as the culprit of cardiovascular diseases and considered a chronic ailment of the aging population, no one suspected how long it took for these plaques to form. When military pathologists studied young U.S. soldiers killed in battle in the Korean War, their results shocked

4

the medical community. More than three-quarters of the soldiers, whose average age was twenty-two, had gross evidence of heart disease. A study on soldiers in the Vietnam War produced similar results. More shocking still was that the Korean soldiers had much less evidence of heart disease.[5]

> Today's procedures are little more than sophisticated plumbing jobs that bypass a blockage but leave the disease intact.

Today, heart disease is a worldwide problem and one of the most serious threats to health in America. Of thirty-five countries surveyed in 1991, U.S. deaths from cardiovascular disease ranked seventeenth for both men and women. The highest death rates were in the Soviet Union, Romania, Poland, Bulgaria, Hungary and Czechoslovakia. The lowest were in Japan, France, Spain, Switzerland and Canada.[6]

More than twenty-six hundred deaths occur in the U.S. each day from cardiovascular disease—one death every thirty-three seconds.[7]

Heart disease deaths kill more people than the next seven causes of death combined. In 1997, it claimed 953,110 lives—an astonishing 41.2 percent of all deaths. Compare that to cancer, which claimed 539,377 deaths; accidents, which claimed 95,644; and HIV (AIDS), which claimed 16,516.[8]

Nearly one of every 2.4 deaths in the U.S. is caused by cardiovascular disease. The cost of cardiovascular disease in 1999 is estimated at $286.5 billion.[9]

And heart disease is not just an "old person's" disease. About one-sixth of all people killed by heart disease annually are under age sixty-five.[10] At least fifty-eight million people in America are suffering right now from some form of heart disease.[11]

AN EQUAL OPPORTUNITY KILLER

The perception that heart disease is a "man's disease" simply is not true. Studies have focused more often on heart disease among men than among women. But studies in recent years that have focused on the impact of heart disease among women found that it has become an equal opportunity killer.

The statistics are clear. Of all females aged forty-five through sixty-four, one in seven suffers some form of heart disease. Of the same aged males, one in six suffers.[12] Of all the people who died of heart disease in 1996, 52.7 percent were women.[13]

While it is true that generally men begin suffering from heart disease at a younger age than women—approximately ten years earlier—more than half the women alive today will die from cardiovascular disease.[14] One in three women above age sixty-five has some form of heart disease.[15]

In 1994, heart disease claimed the lives of four hundred ninety-eight thousand women. Breast cancer claims the lives of about forty-three thousand women per year. Of all female deaths, 44 percent are from heart disease.[16]

Even worse is that heart attacks appear to be much more deadly to women. Women who have heart attacks are twice as likely as men to die within the following two weeks.[17] Forty-four percent of women—compared to 27 percent of men—will die within one year of a heart attack.[18]

A SUFFERING HEART

If you tie a ribbon tightly on the base of any of your fingers, your finger will first change color from red to purple. Before long it will become pale, at which point the pain will be very sharp. The same thing happens to your heart during a myocardial ischemic attack—better known as a heart attack.

Let's take a closer look at why heart attacks occur and why they are so dangerous.

Many different types of heart disease exist, some affecting the valves of the heart, some the walls of the heart and some the chambers—but the most prevalent heart disease involves the coronary arteries—those vessels that feed the heart itself.

> More than half the women alive today will die from cardiovascular disease.

To put it simply, heart disease occurs when inflammation and plaque buildup block coronary arteries, causing reduced or stopped blood flow to the heart.

Arteries are supposed to be flexible and smooth, expanding and contracting as the blood flows through. Nearly all coronary artery disease results from atherosclerosis, which comes from the Greek words *athero,* meaning "porridge or paste," and *sclerosis,* meaning "hardness."[19] With atherosclerosis, deposits of fats and calcium build up on the inner walls. These fat and calcium deposits are called *plaques.*[20]

When these hard plaques damage the inner layer of the artery wall—causing them to harden, thicken and lose elasticity—*arteriosclerosis* occurs. These terms can be confusing

7

terms, so as you go through this book just keep this in mind: *Arteriosclerosis* and *atherosclerosis,* even though they are not synonyms, for all practical purposes mean hardening of the arteries.

> If you tie a ribbon tightly on the base of any of your fingers, before long it will become pale, at which point the pain will be very sharp. The same thing happens to your heart during a heart attack.

Plaque is like the flaky rust inside of an old water pipe. Building up layer by layer, it can eventually block an artery completely and stop the blood flow, or it can narrow an artery and reduce blood flow enough to form a blood clot, or a thrombus. When a blood clot blocks a coronary artery, a heart attack occurs.[21]

We normally think of atherosclerosis in terms of the heart, but it can seriously impact other parts of the body, too. For instance, a diseased carotid artery leading to the brain can cause a stroke. A blocked renal artery leading to the kidney can cause high blood pressure. Atherosclerosis in the arteries leading to the bowel can cause abdominal pain, weight loss or death of the bowels.

Blockage in the arteries supplying the legs with blood can cause difficulty in walking due to muscle discomfort after walking and can eventually lead to leg ulcers and even gangrene.[22]

All of these symptoms are cause by ischemia, or lack of blood, and thus lack of oxygen.

BE AWARE OF THE SYMPTOMS

A coronary artery that fails to send enough blood to the heart muscle causes chest pain, which doctors call *angina pectoris.* *Angina* means "pain," and *pectoris* means "chest."

This pain, often described as a feeling of pressure or heaviness, is usually located in the center of the chest, but it may occur only in the neck, shoulder, arm or lower jaw, particularly on the left side.[23] This pain almost always occurs after the heart has been "stressed" in some way, either by physical activity, emotional stress, cold temperatures—or even after a third helping of pork ribs, French fries, coleslaw and corn on the cob. Anything that increases the heart's workload increases the danger for someone whose coronary arteries are blocked.

If your chest discomfort lasts for less than five seconds or more than twenty minutes, then you are probably not having heart problems (provided it's not a heart attack). If you experience a sharp or "stabbing" pain that is brought on by a sudden movement or deep breath, it's probably not your heart. If your chest pain is confined to a small area, or if it's relieved by rest or by stopping your physical activity, it's probably not your heart (again, provided you are not having a heart attack). In addition, if your chest wall is tender to the touch, it is probably not your heart.[24]

One of the difficulties in diagnosing heart problems is that many of its symptoms are similar to symptoms of less serious afflictions. Signs of a blocked coronary artery can be:

- Indigestion
- Nausea

9

- Abdominal bloating
- Belching
- Vomiting
- Severe pain in the upper right abdomen
- Discomfort unrelated to eating
- Shortness of breath
- Sweating
- Pain radiating to the jaw, neck or arm
- Severe pressure, fullness, squeezing, pain and/or discomfort in the center of the chest that lasts for more than a few minutes
- Clammy skin
- Paleness
- Dizziness or fainting
- Unexplained weakness or fatigue
- Rapid or irregular pulse

Few people jump to the conclusion that they are having a heart attack when they have indigestion or nausea. But identifying the cumulative symptoms could save your life and your quality of life.

THE FINAL DROP

The deathblow of cardiovascular disease is the heart attack, which happens suddenly, but which is caused by years and decades of unhealthy habits. The circumstances surrounding a heart attack are like the one drop of liquid that makes the full glass overflow. That particular drop is not the real problem. The real problem resulted from all of the other drops that went into the glass before it.

Doctors call it acute myocardial infarction, or acute MI.

Myocardial refers to the cardiac muscle or the wall of the heart. Infarction refers to what happens to that wall—the death of the muscle tissue due to lack of oxygen.[25]

A heart attack occurs when the supply of blood to the heart is reduced or stopped because of an inflamed or blocked coronary artery. When the blood stops flowing, the muscle cells become starved for oxygen and begin to die. If enough heart muscle cells die, the victim dies, too. But if enough cells survive, the victim can recover, albeit with a damaged heart.

> Few people jump to the conclusion that they are having a heart attack when they have indigestion or nausea. But identifying the cumulative symptoms could save your life and your quality of life.

How severe a heart attack is depends on several factors, the first of which is the area of the heart that is deprived of oxygen. A person can die when as little as 10 percent of the heart is damaged if the affected area is critical to the heart's ability to function. However, in other cases a victim can survive with damage to 30 to 40 percent of the heart when the affected areas are less critical.[26]

How severe a heart attack is also depends on which coronary artery is blocked. Blockages of some coronary arteries are more life-threatening than others.[27]

At least two hundred fifty thousand people die of heart

attacks each year before they ever reach a hospital. Half of all heart attack victims wait more than two hours before getting help, which is why knowing the warning signs is so critical.[28]

> The deathblow of cardiovascular disease is the heart attack, which happens suddenly, but which is caused by years and decades of unhealthy habits.

Those who survive heart attacks have vastly reduced heart-pumping power. After an attack, the heart struggles to provide the necessary power to move the blood through the blood vessels. The arteries become like a congested freeway when the number of lanes are insufficient to handle all the cars. The heart is overtaken by a disease simply called *congestive heart failure*. This means the heart simply cannot keep up with the demand.

WHAT CAUSES HEART DISEASE?

Hardening of the arteries, or arteriosclerosis, is an inevitable part of the aging process. No one is immune to some form of it. However, for some, the process is more rapid than for others.[29]

What causes heart disease? I believe the most important factors are lifestyle habits—what we eat, whether or not we exercise, if we smoke and so on. However, this is still a subject of controversy in the medical community, and nobody claims to know for certain what all the factors are. But some habits and symptoms have been identified as risk factors:

12

- High blood pressure
- Smoking
- Heavy drinking
- Diabetes
- Genetic makeup
- Poor diet
- Inactivity
- Obesity
- Higher-than-normal levels of cholesterol
- Periodontal disease

EQUAL OPPORTUNITY RISK?

While most of the causes of heart disease apply to both men and women, women have several unique or distinct risk factors. Let's take a look at them.

BIRTH CONTROL PILLS

Oral contraceptives can increase the risk of heart disease for some women, possibly by increasing cholesterol levels and raising blood pressure.[30] When a large number of oral contraceptive users took part in a study, some of them experienced a rise in blood pressure levels. Nevertheless, most of the women remained within the normal range. Just a small percentage of women saw their blood pressure rise to higher levels.[31] This means that oral contraceptives could increase the risk of heart disease for some women.

PREGNANCY

Pregnancy causes major changes in a woman's circulatory system. The volume or amount of a blood in a pregnant woman's body increases by as much as 40 percent. This forces

13

her heart to work much harder to push all that blood through her body. For healthy women, the effect of pregnancy upon the heart is of no more consequence than mild exercise. But for women with underlying heart disease, pregnancy may aggravate those problems.[32]

WOMEN AND OBESITY

For years we have known that obesity and heart disease go hand in hand in men. However, being even mildly overweight can increase a woman's heart attack risk dramatically, perhaps more than in men, according to an eight-year study from Brigham and Women's Hospital in Boston. For example, a woman five feet four and one-half inches tall, who weighs one hundred thirty-seven to one hundred forty-five pounds, increases her risk by 30 percent over a woman the same height who weighs less than one hundred twenty-five pounds.

In women who are approximately 30 percent or more over ideal weight, 70 percent of all heart attacks could be traced to obesity.[33]

DIABETES

Diabetes is a risk factor for heart disease in both men and women because high blood sugar speeds up hardening of the arteries. Nevertheless, researchers have learned that diabetic women have lower "good" cholesterol levels than diabetic men. This is why diabetes increases the risk of a second heart attack in women, but not in men. The reasons for this difference in the sexes are unknown.[34]

WORKING WOMEN

Another study has shown that female clerical workers

have a higher rate of heart attack than homemakers. It seems reasonable to say that the stress of working and balancing home and office may raise blood pressure, cut out exercise time and cause women to eat unhealthy fast foods.[35]

Middle-aged female clerical workers, who usually tend to be sedentary outside of work and to carry excess body weight, have a greater risk of heart attacks and strokes. The reason for this is that they are more likely to have fatty buildup in their carotid arteries—the arteries that carry blood to the head—than women who work in blue-collar and white-collar jobs and other women who do not work outside the home. Carotid artery disease is considered an indicator of risk for heart disease and stroke.[36]

SURVIVING HEART ATTACKS

As previously noted, women who have heart attacks are less likely to survive than men. In addition, nearly 1 percent fewer women than men survive balloon angioplastic surgery. Of those who do, more women than men have reclogging of the arteries, chest pain and other complications.

Bypass surgery is nearly twice as deadly for women. And, after leaving the hospital following a heart attack, a woman is more likely to die of a heart attack than is a man.[37]

BODY SIZE

Body size seems to be a primary factor for why women have heart attacks. One study found that women five feet tall and shorter experience a 50 percent greater chance of having a heart attack than women five feet four inches tall and taller. Some doctors theorize that short women have smaller arteries that clog more easily.

Also, taller women have lower blood cholesterol than

15

shorter ones. This is not the case with men, and the reason for it is uncertain.[38]

WOMEN AND SMOKING

Women are 50 percent more likely than men to suffer a heart attack as a result of smoking, according to a study of more than twenty-four thousand Danish men and women.

Researchers tallied the number of study participants who suffered a fatal or nonfatal heart attack over a twelve-year period. They discovered that the risk of heart attack rose with increased smoking for both men and women. However, the risks were consistently higher for female smokers than for their male counterparts.

It's possible that components of smoke may interact with estrogen.[39]

We will discuss keys to successfully combat each risk factor a little later on, but first let's look at how heart disease is treated. You may even begin to feel the wonderment I experienced when I first looked at this incredibly marvelous machine—your own beating heart.

Chapter 2

Treating
Heart Disease

B ob, a forty-year-old distant cousin of mine, is the father of three, an active member of his church and a rising star in his company. He has finally hit his stride, and all aspects of his life are a joy, but looming over him like an ancient shadow is his family's history of heart disease. All known male members of the family, going back for as many generations as they can think of, have died of a heart attack before they reached age fifty.

When Bob was just twelve, his father died at age forty-five. His grandfather died of a second heart attack at age forty-eight after barely surviving the first one.

Two of his three uncles died of heart attacks; one was forty, and the other was forty-five. The healthiest one had no signs of heart trouble, but died in a car accident at age forty-nine. It is difficult to blame Bob for believing that this pathology is more than hereditary. He is convinced that his family has been cursed with heart disease.

Bob feels that each passing year brings him closer to what

he visualizes as the red zone—the place of imminent danger. When he was in his twenties, the danger seemed far removed. During his thirties, Bob continued to push the issue out of his mind. Now that he has passed the threshold into his forties, he sees himself at the brink of the fated moment when he will collapse to the floor, gasping as his crying wife calls the ambulance.

> Rather than making life changes to avoid heart disease, men and women choose to "cross that bridge when they come to it," not realizing that they are crossing the bridge now and someday it will collapse underneath them.

Bob has seen his doctor several times to talk about heart disease. His physician recommended some minor modifications to his lifestyle, including drugs to lower his cholesterol. But for Bob, nothing can be done but to wait for his future heart problems to strike and hope that he will fare better than his ancestors.

He confided to me, "They didn't have the advantages of ultramodern technology, super heart specialists or the means that I have at my disposal to restore my heart."

Bob has read about how doctors insert a small balloon through an artery in the groin and drag off the plaque that builds up in the arteries. He knows about the stents they can place in the arteries around the heart. He has learned about the small "Roto-rooter" device that grinds the plaque away.

And of course, there is always the ultimate option of having bypass surgery, which Bob sees as so routine as to be harmless.

Having such a marvelous array of technological options at his disposal makes Bob feel more secure, and he talks as if every problem he might face could have a quick and easy solution. He is dazzled by the idea of small gadgets cleaning out his arteries, and he marvels at how science has taken the danger out of heart disease.

"When it hits, I know the doctors will be ready," he often tells his wife.

Bob's approach is typical. Rather than making life changes to avoid heart disease, men and women choose to "cross that bridge when they come to it," not realizing that they are crossing the bridge now and someday it will collapse underneath them.

THE MECHANIC MIND-SET

Many, if not most, patients look to technology first and foremost for answers. Who wouldn't be impressed with what doctors can do nowadays? We treat doctors like mechanics, waiting until we come down with an illness or pain to visit them. We buy cars that don't need their first scheduled tune-ups until one hundred thousand miles, and we expect our bodies to behave the same way.

The reason for this attitude toward coronary disease is a misconception that heart attacks appear suddenly. It is true that heart attacks are sudden, but they represent the culmination of a disease that takes many, many years to develop. There are reports of arteriosclerosis in children as young as three years of age; most American teenagers already suffer, in various degrees, with hardening of the arteries.

19

Most of us know some of the terms and technologies of heart disease from reading the newspaper or from the experience of somebody we know. The explosion of knowledge in the twentieth century shed light on every aspect of the heart and human body. Science has provided so many answers that the average individual knows more about the human body than the greatest thinkers throughout most of history. Fourth graders around the world might astonish Aristotle or Galen with the breadth and exactness of their knowledge of different organs, even if that knowledge was as old as their fourth grade textbooks!

Thanks to modern science, we now know the physical makeup of this fascinating, intricate and wonderful "pump" that forms the vital core of all of our body's functions.

> Many, if not most, patients look to technology first and foremost for answers. Who wouldn't be impressed with what doctors can do nowadays? We treat doctors like mechanics, waiting until we come down with an illness or pain to visit them.

THE SHAPE OF THE HEART

Hold your hand up and make a fist. Look at it closely. That is about the size of your heart. As a child you could have done the same thing and discovered the size of your heart then. The heart grows at the same rate as the fist, so at every stage of development, from birth through adulthood, we can determine the precise size of our heart by looking at our fist.

In the early stages of fetal development, however, the size of the heart relative to body size is nine times greater than when the baby is born. It would be like having a basketball inside your chest! In the weeks after conception a baby's heart occupies most of the baby's midsection. If you have ever seen an ultrasound of a child *in utero,* you probably noticed how the baby is hunched over a large, pulsing heart.

Put your hand on the left side of your rib cage or on the underside of your wrist. As usual, your heart is pumping away, probably at sixty to seventy times per minute. Our hearts beat fastest when we are infants, about one hundred twenty beats per minute. That is because our blood is carrying large amounts of oxygen to our bodies to support our rapid growth. As we become children, our heart slows to about ninety beats per minute, and when we become adults it levels off at seventy to eighty beats. As we reach our retirement years, our hearts slow even further, to about fifty to sixty-five beats per minute.[1]

The human heart is hollow, with four chambers and distinct left and right sides. It weighs about eleven ounces, or less than a can of soda, and pumps unceasingly until the day we die (or until it is replaced with a transplanted heart).

All mammals have four-chambered hearts, from the smallest shrew to the largest whale. In fact, a blue whale's heart is about the size of a Volkswagen Beetle and beats five to six times per minute normally, and three times per minute when it dives deep into the ocean. A blue whale's circulatory system contains ten tons of blood, compared to about 1.3 gallons in the human body. A shrew, on the other hand, has a much smaller heart and a much more rapid heart beat of twelve hundred times per minute.[2]

Interestingly, however, humans and animals share many diseases such as cancer and arthritis, but heart disease is uniquely human. It is virtually unknown in the animal kingdom. Birds and groundhogs never die of clogged arteries or heart attacks.

WITH EVERY BEAT OF YOUR HEART

The heart is located in the middle of our chest inside a structure that is built like a bank vault, making it very difficult to get to. It sits in a moist cavity right between the lungs and behind our breastbone. Surrounding it is the rib cage, and on the bottom is a tough layer of muscle called the diaphragm—the muscle that contracts when we cough. It is difficult to imagine a sturdier "room" for our heart to carry out its business. There, protected from all but the most severe blows, the heart beats one hundred fifteen thousand times per day, forty-two million times per year and more than three billion times in a lifetime.[3]

How does the heart beat? How does it know when to slow down or speed up? The heart is simply a muscle, though clearly our most important one. All muscles tighten and loosen in response to electrical impulses given by the nervous system, which controls the flow of electricity in our bodies. If you have ever touched a live wire and received a shock, you probably felt your muscles tighten involuntarily. When someone touches a high-voltage wire, the hand usually tightens around the wire, making it impossible to let go, which is why, if the voltage is strong enough, he gets electrocuted.

Some muscles, such as those in our arms and legs, function only when we tell them to. But others, such as the lungs, digestive system and heart, function involuntarily. We never have to think about making our hearts beat—and thank God for that.

A heartbeat begins with an electrical impulse sent from a small mass of tissue called the sinus node, which is located on the upper right side of the heart. That impulse causes the heart to contract, first in the top portion and then in the bottom portion a millisecond later. The purpose of the delayed or uneven beat is so the blood moves from the upper chambers into the lower chambers and then out. The heart pushes out 2.5 ounces of blood with every beat. The nervous system tells the heart to pump faster during physical activity and slower during sleep.

> Humans and animals share many diseases such as cancer and arthritis, but heart disease is uniquely human.

The cells in the heart know how to beat in unison. If you place two live heart cells in a petri dish, they will synchronize their beats. If they didn't, each cell would beat at a different time and the heart would accomplish nothing.

The poisons in some wild animals use this to advantage. The sea wasp, a jellyfish native to the waters of Australia and the Philippines, is considered the most deadly creature on earth.[4] Its poison is seven hundred times more powerful than its better-known cousin, the Portuguese man-of-war, and it can paralyze a swimmer's heart in thirty seconds. It is believed that the poison's deadly power to paralyze comes from making the heart's cells beat randomly rather than in unison.

23

So the heart is fist-sized, weighs a little less than a can of soda and beats continuously at the direction of the nervous system.

A MIGHTY ENGINE

Your heart's purpose is to keep a constant flow of oxygen and nutrients going into the body and a constant flow of carbon dioxide and wastes out.

Like the generator at a power plant, the heart is the mighty engine that keeps the rest of the body running. To fully accomplish its purpose, it must feed three parts of the body:

- The body
- The lungs
- Itself

The first involves the circulatory system, the second the pulmonary system and the third the coronary system. Each system is absolutely essential for life.

Systemic circulation

The circulatory system looks like the roots of a tree that start large and become increasingly smaller. Blood is carried by a series of flexible pipes called blood vessels. These perform the same function as the hoses that water your garden. Altogether, an adult body contains nearly sixty thousand miles of blood vessels.

Arteries carry blood away from the heart. Veins run parallel to the arteries and carry blood back to the heart. Capillaries lie in between. Let's look at each.

The blood's journey through the body begins in the *arteries*. When the heart contracts, it sends blood out through the main tube, a large artery called the dorsal aorta, which quickly branches off into smaller arteries and sends blood throughout the body.

Arteries are made of three plies of material: an outer layer of tissue, a middle layer of muscle and a smooth inner wall that allows the blood to flow freely. It is vitally important that they are flexible, smooth on the inside and equipped with muscles that help move the blood along. The muscles in the artery walls actually pump in counter-rhythm with the heart, contracting when the heart relaxes. The blood in the arteries is bright red, meaning that it is full of oxygen.

Capillaries are the microscopic vessels that connect arteries to veins. They are so small that blood can only pass through them one cell at a time. The blood cells release oxygen through the capillary walls and into the tissue, and the tissue passes carbon dioxide through the wall and into the blood cells. In a sense, the blood cells first deliver the groceries, then take out the trash.

> Your heart's purpose is to keep a constant flow of oxygen and nutrients going into the body and a constant flow of carbon dioxide and wastes out.

Capillaries also help the body to release heat. When the body temperature rises, as during exercise or a hot shower, the blood rushes heat into the capillaries, which quickly release heat into the tissue, dispersing it and maintaining a constant body temperature.

25

Veins are thinner-walled vessels that lack the muscles and strength of the arteries. After the exchange of gases in the tissues, capillaries carry blood into the veins so it can be routed back to the heart. If you could look at it, you would see that this blood is dark purple, which indicates a lack of oxygen.

To keep the blood from going backwards or pooling, veins are equipped with valves that open and close to keep blood moving forward. They are like doorways, or the levels on a fish ladder.

THE PULMONARY SYSTEM

One of blood's main tasks is to bring oxygen to the body, and that is why it must pass through the lungs. When purplish, waste-filled blood arrives in the heart, it is immediately pumped into the lungs. There the blood cells let go of carbon dioxide and grab oxygen. The blood then goes back into the heart, where it is pumped through the dorsal aorta and begins its circuit again.

THE CORONARY SYSTEM

While feeding the rest of the body, the heart must also feed itself. The heart can store nutrients, but it needs a constant supply of oxygen. About 5 percent of the blood pumped by the heart goes to feed the heart muscle.[5]

Two main coronary arteries and their branches, ranging in size from one-fifth to one-eighth of an inch, form a crown of vessels around the top of the heart that supply it with blood.[6] The word *crown* in Latin is *corona*, hence *coronary vessels*. In a normal heart, these arteries give the heart a continuous supply of oxygen.

But when they are blocked off, the heart begins to run

short on nutrients and oxygen, and the heart begins to "fail." Before long, this can lead to a heart attack.

DIAGNOSING AND
TREATING HARD ARTERIES

Physicians have many ways of feeling, hearing, measuring and even seeing blockages in your arteries. Doctors can feel for a pulse in an area they believe is afflicted. Usually the more advanced the arteriosclerosis, the less pulse can be felt in a given area.

As the artery becomes blocked, it can actually create noise that sounds like water roaring over rocky rapids. Your physician can listen to this noise and use special equipment to measure the amount of blood going to a specific area of the body.[7]

Today, doctors use several common procedures to diagnose and treat arteriosclerosis. To find the best therapy for you, it is important to get a qualified diagnosis. Modern technology has made unimaginable recent advances to help you.

Computerized, digital images can precisely map out any and all arteries in your body. Recently, the Oasis of Hope hospital acquired the most advanced computerized machinery available to make the most accurate diagnoses. Our very powerful software now makes it possible to view calcifications within the coronary arteries while avoiding the dangers of some of the more invasive techniques.

Let's take a closer look at some of these stunning medical technologies that can help diagnose and treat heart disease.

LOCATING BLOCKED ARTERIES

You saw one method of locating arterial blockages at the beginning of the book in my father's situation. This mapping of the arteries, also called coronary arteriography, is done using a procedure called cardiac catheterization.

During this procedure, a doctor guides a thin plastic tube through an artery in the arm or leg and into the coronary arteries. Then the doctor injects a liquid dye through the catheter. The dye is visible in x-rays, which record the course of the dye as it flows through the arteries.

> In the U.S. alone, about 700,000 angioplasties are performed nationwide each year.

By mapping the dye's flow, the doctor identifies blocked areas. Once the mapping is completed, the doctor can decide the best course of action.[8] Also during the catheterization, a small sample of heart tissue can be obtained for abnormalities to be examined later under the microscope.

ECHOCARDIOGRAPHY

Another way to map the heart is through echoes. Pulses are sent into the chest, and high-frequency sound waves bounce off of the heart's walls and valves. The returning echoes are electronically plotted to produce a picture of the heart called an echocardiogram.[9]

Of course, once your physician has determined where your arteries are blocked, then he or she may recommend several treatment options. Let's take a brief look at some of the medical options available to those suffering from heart disease.

ANGIOPLASTY

If your doctor prescribes an invasive procedure called an

angioplasty, this is what you can expect. A doctor will insert and guide a catheter toward the blocked area of the artery. Then a second catheter with a small balloon on the tip will be passed through the first catheter.

Once the balloon tip reaches the blocked area, the balloon will be inflated, pressing down the plaque buildup and widening the artery so that blood can flow freely. Finally, the balloon will be deflated and removed, and a stent—or a tiny expandable metal coil—may be placed inside the artery to keep it open. As we will see, this kind of invasive procedure is used routinely to prevent heart attacks.[10]

A second version of this procedure is called an *atherectomy,* in which the blocked area inside the artery is "shaved" away by a tiny device on the end of a catheter. In a third version of this procedure, lasers actually "vaporize" the blockage in the artery.[11]

It was not until the 1970s that the first angioplasty was performed on people. In 1997, more than one million angioplasties were performed worldwide, making it the most common medical intervention in the world.[12] In the U.S. alone, about seven hundred thousand angioplasties are performed nationwide each year.[13]

HEART BYPASS SURGERY

For some, your doctor may suggest having a coronary artery bypass graft surgery. Here, a surgeon takes a healthy blood vessel from another part of the body (usually the leg or inside the chest wall) and uses it to construct a detour around the blocked coronary artery. One end of the vessel is grafted, or attached, right below the blockage while the other end is grafted right above the blockage. As a result, enough blood can flow to the heart muscle again.

In a double bypass surgery, two grafts are performed. In a triple bypass, three grafts. In a quadruple, four grafts.[14]

HEART TRANSPLANT

The most radical surgical possibility is a transplant of the heart or of the part of the heart that is needed.

When a healthy person dies, his or her heart can still be used. The heart patient's diseased heart is removed, and the healthy donor heart is then attached. The operation is extremely complicated by many blood vessels that must be detached and then reattached.

During the operation, the patient is connected to a heart and lung machine that keeps his blood circulating. After the operation, a risk remains that the patient may reject the new heart. Tissue types have to be matched perfectly for the transplant to be successful. As a result, the number of transplants performed is quite low.

One last medical intervention is left—the artificial heart. Let's investigate.

> When given the choice between preventive maintenance and a wait-and-see approach, we choose to wait because technology feels as if it has taken the sting out of any problems that may arise.

30

ARTIFICIAL HEART

Artificial hearts mimic the action of real hearts, but they are not viable options for long-term survival. Nevertheless, they can help a patient survive until a donor heart is available.

The most well-known procedure involving an artificial heart took place in 1982 when a "Jarvik-7" artificial heart was implanted into a patient named Barney Clark. For various medical reasons, a transplant operation was not an option for Clark. He survived with the Jarvik-7 for one hundred twelve days.[15]

Very recently, a new kind of artificial heart has been approved for limited use. It is the first implanted heart to be tested in eighteen years. This new heart is the size of a softball and is entirely self-contained (the Jarvik-7 was connected to a pump the size of a washing machine). It is made of titanium, plastic and silicone fluid, and it pumps blood through the body just as a natural heart does. An implanted battery is continually recharged using radio waves that transfer electricity from an external battery. The internal battery allows the person to function for half an hour without outside electricity. A small computer worn on a belt pack receives data from sensors inside the heart that tell the heart when to pump more or less.[16]

These procedures are a few of the more common wonders of modern technology. Being graced with one hundred twelve more days was no doubt a wonderful blessing for Barney Clark. But how much better for Barney and all of the other millions who suffer if heart disease could be bypassed completely.

To even consider such a notion, we will have to change the way we think. Too many of us are just like my distant cousin who placed all of this trust in technology. I believe there is a better way. But this better way begins by rethinking our attitudes about modern medicine.

THE DOC MECHANIC

When given the choice between preventive maintenance and a wait-and-see approach, we choose to wait because technology feels as if it has taken the sting out of any problems that may arise.

And why not have this attitude? Many of us think that one day we have all sorts of trouble because our heart is not getting enough blood; the next we are fit, functioning human beings, all because of our visit to the surgery room. Voilá! We shake the doctor's hand and walk out, pondering the wonderful times in which we live.

But it is imperative that we begin taking responsibility for our own physical well-being and stop irresponsibly depositing this task on doctors. Physicians can do much for us, but only through our efforts and discipline can we avoid and even reverse the hardening of our arteries.

In addition, modern technology is marvelous, but it may not be exactly all it's cracked up to be. Before we make up our minds, let's investigate a little further to determine if we want to live completely at the mercy of technology.

Chapter 3

At the Mercy
of Technology

I am a surgeon, and after twenty years of working side by side with my father, I have learned that surgery, even to save a life, should be used as a last resort.

Following my father's heart procedure, he was helped off of the gurney and allowed to dress and return home to await the results. It wasn't long before we learned how grave his situation really was. The doctors warned that without immediate heart bypass surgery, he would die a terrible and suffocating death within months. All of his main coronary arteries were severely constricted, and the flow of blood was deficient to the heart muscle. To restore my father's blood flow to his heart muscle, the doctors recommended seven bypasses. This made sense in light of his angiography, they said.

I am from three generations of surgeons; my family founded the Oasis of Hope hospital and has been a forerunner of much of the medical thought that is receiving ever-widening acceptance around the world. Nevertheless, after learning the outcome of this heart procedure, my father determined not to have surgery.

This does not mean that I am always against surgery, but the surgical approach must make sense in light of the facts of the particular case and *never* be a first option. If your experience is anything like my father's, you may be surprised to learn that surgery is not the only option—and it may not be the best option, either. As a matter of fact, in many situations it isn't a good option at all. In this chapter, I want to evaluate the limitations and shortcomings of modern heart treatments in the light of scientific findings to help you become better informed.

THE DIFFICULTIES OF
DIAGNOSING HEART DISEASE

Doctors, even with ultramodern machinery, still have a difficult time diagnosing heart disease because its symptoms, signs and anatomy can vary so widely.

One author writes:

> Persons with extensive lesions in their coronary artery do not necessarily suffer from angina [pain]. For many, the first warning symptom of coronary heart disease is a heart attack. Why an insufficient supply of blood produces sharp pains in some individuals and no symptoms in others remains a major unsolved mystery...For the unwary physician, angina can be easily confused with anxiety, hyperventilation, heartburn, ulcers and inflammation of the gallbladder.[1]

My father-in-law, who also had a heart attack, suffered for two months with nausea and loss of appetite and lost twenty-five pounds before his doctor discovered that he had had a heart attack and was having an aberrant type of angina.

The Framingham study, which observed more than ten thousand people over a thirty-year observation period, showed that one-fourth of the heart attacks suffered were not recognized or treated. In half of those cases, the victim did not seek medical care.[2] Surprisingly, fatal heart attacks are more often the ones that are overlooked, rather than mild ones. This prompted the study's author to write, "The failure to diagnose 47 percent of fatal acute myocardial infarctions [fatal heart attacks] was appalling."[3]

If you do recognize your symptoms as a heart attack and show up at the emergency room of a hospital, you won't necessarily receive an accurate diagnosis even then. Two in eight people who suffered a heart attack and went to the hospital were sent home. Additionally, 40 percent of those admitted to the hospital for chest pains did not have heart disease.[4]

> Once a heart attack comes upon you, the damage has already been done. No one should completely rely on after-the-fact medical care to "cure" him or her of heart disease.

Tragically, even if your heart attack is correctly diagnosed and treated, the death of heart tissue is not reversible. Once a heart attack comes upon you, the damage has already been done. No one should completely rely on after-the-fact medical care to "cure" him or her of heart disease.

In 1977, in lieu of the study presented to the U.S. Senate on *Dietary Goals for the United States*, Dr. Beverly Winikoff of the Rockefeller Foundation warned, "There is a widespread and unfounded confidence in the ability of medical science to cure or mitigate the effects of such diseases once they occur... There is, in reality, very little that medical science can do..." Dr. Winikoff then appealed that "appropriate public education must emphasize the unfortunate but clear limitations of current medical practice in curing the common killer diseases." In spite of the tremendous advances since then, this statement holds true today.

> Few doctors even consider less invasive methods of treatment. However, when invasive and noninvasive treatments were compared to one another in a study, the results were astonishing.

THE RISKS OF TREATMENTS

More treatment and more invasive treatments are not always better, and they are often fatal. Recently a doctor wrote in the *New England Journal of Medicine (NEJM)*:

> The authors and reporters [of a particular study] failed to mention the potential complications of catheterization and the possibility of overtreatment (i.e., unnecessary catheterization). In fact, there is growing evidence

that more treatment is not always better and can actually be harmful. A study recently reported in the *Journal,* for example, found that an invasive strategy (immediate cardiac catheterization) for all patients with a non−Q-wave myocardial infarction [heart attack] resulted in higher rates of myocardial infarction [heart attack] and death than a conservative approach. [They] undoubtedly recognized that referring a patient for catheterization is not always the right decision.[5]

OVERTESTING THE HEART

Dramatic risks are involved whenever you use invasive tests and treatments. Yet, many doctors order too many seriously dangerous tests to deal with their doubts, rather than seeking less invasive methods. For many patients, all that would have been needed was a little more time.

Mridu Gulati, M.D., said:

> When it is difficult to establish a diagnosis, the first inclination is often to amass more data by performing increasingly sophisticated tests at the expense of a careful evaluation of the studies that have already been performed. The most important therapeutic intervention for this patient would have been tincture of time.[6]

Doctors and patients today rely heavily on tests, perhaps believing that it is better to be safe than sorry or they are scared of lawsuits for omitting diagnoses. The problem is that these tests, no matter how professionally and technologically glittering, are not void of serious risk.

As we saw earlier, angiography is a method of putting a

catheter into the heart through an artery in the groin or arm, injecting dye into the heart and then taking an x-ray of it so that the crown of arteries is visible. This method, while technologically pleasing and awe-inspiring, can hurt or even kill people. The catheter can clog the heart and provoke a heart attack, which is why a surgical team is required to be present whenever an angiography is performed.

> It is actually possible that millions of these dangerous treatments are being performed every year with questionable benefits.

These dangers are less common now, but is the benefit of angiography significant enough to put any patient at risk?

Few doctors even consider less invasive methods of treatment. However, when invasive and noninvasive treatments were compared to one another in a study, the results were astonishing.

When nine hundred twenty heart attack patients were tracked for nearly two years, with patients randomly divided into two groups and treated either surgically or noninvasively, the less invasively treated patients fared far better. Those who were treated with an invasive strategy had worse outcomes during the first year of follow-up. In addition, the number who died or who had another heart attack was significantly higher in the invasive-strategy group. Therefore, researchers determined that individuals suffering from a heart attack of the type studied do not benefit from routine, early invasive management.[7]

INCREASED RISK?

Some experts believe that having angioplastic surgery actually increases your risk of heart attacks, the need for additional angioplasties and even death. Let's look.

A study published in a prestigious medical journal found that "angioplasty may increase myocardial infarction [heart attack], mortality, or the need for further angioplasty. Clinicians should be restrained in their recommendations for percutaneous transluminal coronary angioplasty, reserving the procedure for patients whose symptoms of angina are not well controlled on medical treatment."[8]

It is actually possible that millions of these dangerous treatments are being performed every year with questionable benefits.

Thomas Moore, a health policy analyst at George Washington University Medical Center and the author of several books critical of the medical industry, writes:

> Millions undergo hazardous treatment of undetermined benefit because the proper controlled studies were never performed. Cardiologists and surgeons became so deeply committed to bypass surgery that they could not appreciate the mounting evidence that the benefits of the procedure were significantly limited. This lack of information has the unintended effect of depriving all patients of the fundamental right of informed consent.[9]

VICE PRESIDENT CHENEY'S HEART TREATMENT

During the 2000 presidential campaign, then-vice-presidential candidate Dick Cheney checked himself into the hospital after suffering a heart attack, and the doctors implanted stents into his coronary arteries. Within days, even hours, he was back on the campaign trail. It seemed that doctors had performed another miracle.

However, the vice president's situation showed the embarrassing side of mainstream heart treatment—the fact that in one in five people who receive stents or other interventional procedures, the artery closes up again, and very rapidly. That, of course, leads to more interventions.

A study published and posted at the website of the National Institutes of Health looked at the success rates of angiography, angioplasty and bypass surgery in six countries: the United States, Australia, Brazil, Canada, Hungary and Poland. They found first that patients in the U.S. and Brazil were far more likely to undergo these invasive treatments because the hospitals had such easy access to the technology. But the startling conclusion was that these procedures did *nothing* to lengthen life. The study reported:

> This relatively aggressive approach led at six months to a more substantial decrease in refractory angina in the United States and Brazil than in Canada and Australia, but no improvement in rates of cardiovascular mortality and MI [heart attack]. There was a significant increase in stroke, and major bleeding events. In concert with findings from other recent randomized trials, the OASIS registry data suggest that although there are fewer hospital re-admissions for unstable angina, there is a trend toward increased rates of death, MI, and stroke. These data urge a cautious approach to the use of invasive procedures in patients with unstable angina

unless future trials demonstrate a clear benefit with an aggressive approach."[10]

Not only did the procedures *not* improve life span, but they seemed to *cause* more strokes and "major bleeding events."

After four different trials found no benefit to invasive surgeries, the *New England Journal of Medicine* commented at length:

> With remarkable clarity and consistency, all four studies show that routine angiography and revascularization do not reduce the incidence of nonfatal reinfarction [second heart attack] or death as compared with the more conservative... approach. In fact, in [one study] the aggressive strategy (which these investigators call 'invasive') was associated with increased mortality during hospitalization, at one month, and at one year.
>
> Although all four trials found that the incidence of adverse events was similar (or greater) in patients whose acute coronary syndromes were managed aggressively than in those assigned to conservative management, an aggressive approach continues to be chosen by most physicians in the United States, whereas a conservative strategy is more likely to be followed in Canada and Europe.
>
> Although the patients enrolled in the United States were more likely than their Canadian counterparts to undergo coronary angiography (68 percent vs. 35 percent, respectively) and subsequent revascularization (31 percent vs. 12 percent), the incidence of reinfarction [second heart attack] and death during more than three

years of follow-up was similar. A strong relation was noted between the availability of angiography in a geographic area and the likelihood that aggressive management would be chosen. However, the increased use of invasive procedures did not reduce the incidence of recurrent infarction or death.

In Europe and Canada, in contrast, patients who… were assigned to conservative management underwent angiography and revascularization one-third to one-half as often as their U.S. counterparts, yet their outcome was similar, and routine aggressive management offered no substantial benefit.[11]

WHY PREFER AGGRESSIVE TREATMENTS?

It may be that some doctors use more aggressive treatments because they want to be seen by the patients as doing everything within their power to cure the heart disease. Some doctors have admitted that they feared lawsuits might result if they didn't pursue the most drastic measures.

Experts admit that research evidence is often ignored when it conflicts with their preconceived notions. For example, the *NEJM* said, "Primary angioplasty for acute myocardial infarction [heart attacks] is widely used and enthusiastically advocated, yet direct comparisons with [other therapies] in relatively small numbers of patients showed, at best, only a small benefit of angioplasty, and larger studies showed none. Many physicians in the United States, even today, continue to believe that all patients with acute coronary syndromes are best treated with prompt coronary angiography and revascularization, despite the absence of scientific support for such an approach."[12]

In addition, the high cost of such procedures has created an economic boon that encourages their use. "[A]s compared with Canada and Europe, the United States has an abundance of facilities for prompt angiography and revascularization, physicians trained to perform these procedures, and monetary remuneration to the facilities and physicians. The combination of these factors encourages the use of angiography and revascularization."[13]

UNNECESSARY BYPASSES?

A wealthy friend of mine went to the cardiologist for a routine heart stress test. He had no symptoms and was leading a normal life. Doctors discovered a spot of the heart muscle that was not receiving a good flow of blood. Immediately he was wheeled off to a catheterization lab where an angiogram showed three very narrow coronary arteries. Now he was whisked off to the operating room for a preventative triple bypass surgery.

The startling conclusion was that these procedures did nothing to lengthen life.

He came out of the surgery feeling wonderful. But he was feeling wonderful before he went under the knife! As any surgeon will tell you, it is gratifying to operate on healthy people because even if you don't fix anything, they come out feeling good.

The problem is that my friend now has a false sense of security. Now he believes that his chances of having a heart attack are small. Therefore, he has not changed his lifestyle

43

habits. It is true that narrowed coronary arteries have a higher risk of closing, or occlusion, but it is debatable that a preventative bypass will be of any value. In fact, bypass surgery may do more harm than good.

To explain this properly I need to mention how the body responds to a narrowing coronary artery. When a coronary artery is narrowed or blocked, the body begins to create other arteries that carry the blood around the blockage. This is like redirecting traffic onto a side street, except that the body is actually constructing new avenues for the blood to flow. This is the body's way of healing itself and providing a natural bypass. Obviously, this process is good for patients who do not have an acute closure of the artery that leads to heart attack. My friend is an example of someone who had narrowing but not acute closure.

Unfortunately, one of the problems with bypass surgery is that it seems to speed up the rate at which affected arteries close up in the days that follow an operation. It also stops the body from creating those "natural bypass" arteries. It is a known fact that the surgery itself harms the artery that is bypassed at the site of where the new vessel is attached to the damaged artery (the anastomosis). The narrowed or blocked arteries can close very suddenly, and the new vessels that bypass them clog very frequently, resulting in a much more serious heart attack.

Howard H. Wayne, a renowned cardiologist, said:

> A major concern is the acceleration of the arteriosclerotic process in the coronary arteries that are treated. For example, vessels that are bypassed often show rapid progression of the occlusive process which led to

the patient's symptoms. More importantly, collateral vessels that had developed over a period of time to compensate for a narrowed artery will usually disappear following bypass surgery. Thus, the ischemic heart muscle may actually be worse off following such surgery. The importance of these collateral vessels is illustrated by the fact that when a coronary artery is severely narrowed, and then becomes completely occluded, it has little effect on cardiac function.[14]

"Because of these facts," Dr. Wayne continues, " the common practice of rushing patients in for emergency or urgent surgery because of a severely narrowed coronary artery is completely unnecessary, and needlessly frightens the patient and his family."[15]

> As any surgeon will tell you, it is gratifying to operate on healthy people because even if you don't fix anything, they come out feeling good.

Am I against heart surgery? No way! It saves many lives. But while bypass surgeries, when judiciously applied, can save your life in a pinch, you must not lose the sight of the fact that they do not *cure* heart disease. Surgeries only bypass a short part of the disease. More research should be aimed at preventing and curing, instead of bypassing, arteriosclerosis.

Bypass surgery appears woefully far from fulfilling its promise of providing a problem-free solution to heart attacks. One observer noted that half of the bypass operations

45

performed in the U.S. are unnecessary. Except in certain well-defined situations, bypass surgery does not save lives or prevent heart attacks.

Another major study found that:

> There was also no long-term survival benefit for high-risk patients assigned to bypass surgery. The probabilities of remaining free of myocardial infarction and of being alive without infarction were significantly higher with initial medical therapy... This trial provides strong evidence that initial bypass surgery did not improve survival for low-risk patients, and that it did not reduce the overall risk of myocardial infarction. Although there was an early survival benefit with surgery in high-risk patients (up to a decade), long-term survival rates became comparable in both treatment groups. In total, there were twice as many bypass procedures performed in the group assigned to surgery without any long-term survival or symptomatic benefit.[16]

Shockingly, bypass operations provided *no long-term survival or symptomatic benefit!* That means life was neither lengthened nor enriched. Such astonishing evidence makes one wonder why on earth bypass surgery remains the cornerstone of heart care.

SPEEDING UP THE DISEASE PROCESS

The heart surgery seems to speed up the rate at which affected arteries close up again and may do more harm than good to the artery.

This was demonstrated in full public view recently when Vice President Dick Cheney had to have more urgent procedures performed after a coronary artery began to close up. It was the same artery that had received a stent less than four months earlier during the campaign. Cheney has suffered four heart attacks in his life, the first when he was only thirty-seven years old. He underwent quadruple bypass surgery in 1988.[17]

> While bypass surgeries, when judiciously applied, can save your life in a pinch, you must not lose the sight of the fact that they do not *cure* heart disease.

It is debatable whether Mr. Cheney would have fared better without the ministrations of modern medicine. It is also quite possible that these procedures may have saved the vice president's life, but I hope that he finally comes to grips with the fact that he needs to do something to stop the atherosclerotic process, not only bypass it. Only lifestyle changes can achieve this.

BYPASSES LOWER MENTAL ACUITY

Thousands of bypasses are performed yearly. These bypasses put people at risk, not only of dying during the process or increasing the advent of more cardiac events, but also their quality of life in the long run can be seriously impaired. Unfortunately, the patient may not be completely aware of it.

It is widely known that patients suffer temporary diminished mental acuity after bypass surgery, possibly because of the flow of blood to the brain during the time the patient is dependent on a heart and lung machine that pumps the blood when the heart is stopped to work on it. Unfortunately, what is temporary for many is an improvement in mental function that later is permanently compromised.

A recent study in the *NEJM* says that five years after having bypass surgeries, 40 percent of the people tested showed a 20 percent drop in mental capacity. In other words, four in ten people lost one-fifth of their brainpower.[18]

STENTS—A BROKEN PROMISE

About half a million people receive coronary stents each year in the U.S. Nevertheless, stents too have not been shown to help people live longer, despite their wide use. Since the introduction of coronary stents into clinical practice in the early 1990s, the number of stent implantations has increased so rapidly that they are currently used in 60 to 70 percent of all interventional procedures.[19]

And while stents had been placed only in larger vessels, doctors have also begun using them in smaller ones as well as technology and skill have improved. But while stents have shown a few short-term benefits, experts admit that they cannot even be sure that stents actually are saving lives.

A recent *NEJM* study said:

> It is disappointing that no study has shown that stents favorably influence mortality; in fact, several trials, including the study by Grines et al., report higher rates of death and myocardial infarction [heart attack] among patients randomly assigned to stent implantation. In all these trials, rates of death and myocardial infarction among patients who received stents were only slightly

and not significantly higher than those among patients who did not, and none of the trials had sufficient power to detect a difference in mortality.

These findings are of prime importance to patients and physicians, and one can only speculate why the placement of an intracoronary stent would not result in a beneficial effect on mortality.[20]

Stents are not lengthening lives. One doctor wrote in the *NEJM:*

> It is disappointing to reflect on how quickly stenting was fully embraced by the cardiology community for the wrong reasons. Unfortunately, in hospitals throughout the United States today, patients…undergo stenting even though there are no data to support these applications. Furthermore, in the case of excellent results with balloon angioplasty, there are no data to show that adding a stent to the dilated segment is necessary or beneficial.

ANGIOGRAMS—ARE THEY TRULY HELPFUL?

The value of angiograms has also come into question. Angiograms help doctors measure the width of coronary arteries, but some observers note that there is only a minor connection between the width of the coronary artery and the patient's overall heart health.

> The vast majority of the total coronary circulation cannot even be seen on an angiogram simply because the angiographic technique is unable to visualize vessels smaller than 0.5 mm…Thus, if the objective of coronary

49

angiograms is to visualize the amount of blood flow to different regions of the heart, it fails miserably.[21]

The study goes on to suggest that angiograms do not provide enough information to help prevent heart attacks.

> Although a single angiogram will tell us if coronary artery disease has been present, it cannot tell us if that disease has become acutely worse, and is the direct cause of the patient's new symptoms, or alternatively, the presence of coronary artery disease is merely coincidental, and there is some other explanation for the patient's symptoms.[22]

We are seeking solutions from machines and chemicals. We want a silver bullet, but none exists.

MY FATHER'S EXAMPLE

To restore my father's blood flow to his heart muscle, the doctors recommended seven bypasses. They felt it made sense in the light of his angiography. But the surgeons did not answer the most important question: Would a bypass operation—which would threaten my father's life—restore the function of my father's heart? Would the damaged heart muscle be revived?

Because in my father's case it would not, he decided the surgery didn't make much sense. Why not? I can explain it best as a picture. No doubt you have seen video footage of little towns affected by hurricanes. Mile after mile of neighborhoods are leveled. Nothing is left standing.

Imagine that those neighborhoods are the cells of the heart muscle. Clearing the streets to allow traffic will do little for the destroyed houses. That is why many times the surgery is worthless. Only when the muscle is alive will the revascularization be very effective.

This mistake happened to my father-in-law. Since he had no typical symptoms, after his heart attack was diagnosed, he underwent angioplasty with stent installment. His condition did not improve as expected, and another angiography was performed to determine if the stent was open. It was. He underwent another test, called a "thallium" test, to determine if the heart's muscle was viable. This test reveals that when the cells have died and become scarred, a bypass operation cannot help.

The test showed that the angioplasty and stent implanted by the surgeons had improved circulation, but to an area that was already dead and scarred. My father-in-law could not benefit from this procedure. It would have created a needless risk.

OVEREMPHASIZING THE PROCEDURE

Technology has done little to stem heart disease. At best Americans appear to be having the same number of heart attacks, but the attacks are less deadly. In other words, the statistics show that even though the number of heart attacks has not changed dramatically, the number of deaths by heart attack has decreased.[23]

At worst, the numbers of deaths are false because of underreporting. A recent study at Yale University indicated differences in the reported cause of death and the cause of death determined by autopsy. When the deaths are corrected to match the autopsy results, today's death rate from heart disease is higher than in the past.[24]

51

THE DRUG MYSTIQUE

Despite the astounding number of drugs that have been developed, we should not fall into the trap of trusting drugs to do what only lifestyle changes can.

Sometimes drugs work well; sometimes they don't. I recently read about a drug called ramipril, which has been shown to reduce the incidence of heart attacks, stroke and death from heart disease.[25] There appear to be no side effects at all. Such drugs can save lives. But even drugs such as ramipril cannot affect the underlying causes of heart disease. At best they put a bandage over the problem.

Heart disease is still such a mystery that to think we can "solve" it with drugs is to welcome unknown problems. For example, drugs are commonly used to lower blood pressure. Doctors prescribe them; patients take them. It is medical orthodoxy that lowering blood pressure will reduce heart disease.

But a recent study in the *NEJM* showed that people with the same levels of blood pressure vary widely in their susceptibility to heart disease.[26] Apparently there is no ideal blood pressure. It is likely that there is a range, but experts cannot agree on what it is.

Does this mean high blood pressure doesn't matter? Absolutely not! Does it mean that we should use caution when prescribing drugs to lower blood pressure? I would say yes. Before we can say that a drug will help, we must better understand the problem. We should know what we want the drug to achieve, why and how many lives we think will be saved with its use.

Should we pump chemicals into many thousands needlessly when the same benefits can be enjoyed through changes in exercise and diet? Rather than first opting for medical intervention, doctors must look at the whole picture. Doctors must learn how a particular person lives to understand his or her risk of heart disease. It's not enough to know his blood pressure or heart size.

Drugs seem to be an easy solution. But are they too easy? Are they the best solution? Is the situation then so hopeless? Certainly not.

In the next chapters I intend to expound on practical, inexpensive and effective practices that I hope will inspire you to make the necessary changes that will help you keep your "ticker" ticking longer, but first, let's clarify some misconceptions and myths.

MY FATHER'S QUALITY OF LIFE

My father underwent an extremely expensive and potentially fatal testing procedure that provided a wonderful diagnosis, but the recommended medical and surgical approach was excessive and, in my father's case, put his life unnecessarily at risk. After careful consideration, he decided that his only real

> A recent study at Yale University indicated differences in the reported cause of death and the cause of death determined by autopsy. When the deaths are corrected to match the autopsy results, today's death rate from heart disease is higher than in the past.

solution involved important lifestyle changes and alternative procedures to cleanse the plaque from his arteries. If he had taken the strictly surgical route, who knows where he would be. But for the past sixteen years he has enjoyed an excellent quality of life after employing vital, heart-smart keys that have given him extended years and added good health.

Let's turn now and take a look at these vital keys for heart health—keys that can make the difference for you, too!

SECTION II
BECOME HEART SMART—
KEYS TO DEVELOPING
OR RECLAIMING
A HEALTHY HEART

Chapter 4

The Stunning Truth About Cholesterol

After a lecture I had been invited to give, my wife and I were people-watching and enjoying a wonderful view of Jackson Square Cathedral in New Orleans, one of America's richest cultural cities. Visit the French Quarter and you will see beautiful architecture, wrought-iron fences and brick streets. A few blocks over is Bourbon Street, home of jazz and the blues (and the country's ungodliest party—Mardi Gras).

We ended our walking tour at a popular café and decided to sit a while and enjoy a sinfully and decidedly unhealthy pastry after a not-so-holy dinner. Dining is a passionate art form in New Orleans, and I reminded myself on that day of what I constantly remind my patients: It is not what you do occasionally but what you do routinely that makes or breaks your healthy lifestyle.

Apparently New Orleaners are routinely tempted by its famous Cajun food, and they succumb to its appealing (or should I say "appalling") pastries. Little wonder that it is also the heart disease capital of the U.S. Studies have shown that heart disease rates in New Orleans and other cities like Chicago, Detroit and New York are significantly higher than throughout the rest of the country.[1]

How ironic that this "cholesterol capital" sits at the mouth of the country's most significant "artery"—the Mississippi River, which fans out into a triangular delta and dumps its fresh water into the Gulf of Mexico. The river is a picture of circulation. As the water travels downstream from the headwaters in Minnesota, it constantly picks up dirt particles. And when the water reaches the river's mouth in New Orleans, that dirt is deposited as sediment.

Sediment is an enemy of free-flowing water. It builds up along the banks and on the river bottom and generally restricts the water's flow. Sediment must be dredged out of the mouths of many rivers so the water can flow freely.

That is a picture of what happens to our arteries. Sediment builds up, restricting blood flow. This is called atherosclerosis, a buildup of plaque in the arteries traditionally linked directly to cholesterol. But is all that you've heard about cholesterol entirely true? Let's find out.

YOUR HEART AND CHOLESTEROL

Although most of us have heard a great deal about this life-impacting substance over the past several years, few really understand the stunning truth about cholesterol. Let's take an in-depth look at this substance that holds enormous power in your body either for good or for disaster.

THE GOOD, THE BAD AND THE UGLY

Cholesterol is now a part of popular healthy heart culture.

Fear of high cholesterol has led many people to stop eating eggs, to take regular cholesterol tests and to consume drugs that lower cholesterol.

Not only do we have good and bad cholesterol, but there is even ugly cholesterol as well. The "good" is called high-density lipoproteins (HDL), the "bad" is called low-density lipoproteins (LDL), and the "ugly" is known as very low-density lipoproteins (VLDL) and the triglycerides, which are extremely low-density lipoproteins.

Cholesterol, or lipids, is found in the blood and is linked directly to heart disease. The word *cholesterol* comes from the Greek *chole,* meaning "bile," and *stereos,* meaning "solid," so called because it was first found in gallstones.

> Cholesterol has a function and a role in our bodies' natural balance and maintenance. It is as normal a part of the human body as enzymes, hormones and blood cells.

Let's look at some facts about cholesterol.

THE FUNCTION OF CHOLESTEROL

Like most Americans, you might know the range that is recommended for "healthy" cholesterol, and you might even be able to visualize what cholesterol does in your arteries. You probably get a picture in your mind of a yellow, oily sludge becoming encrusted on the inside of your artery walls and narrowing the flow of blood. You may imagine that cholesterol comes from fast food and goes directly into your bloodstream.

In reality, cholesterol is not really a fat, as many people believe. It is a pearl-colored, waxy, solid alcohol that feels like soap.[2]

An even bigger surprise is that it is not a foreign intruder introduced by eggs, mayonnaise and drive-through hamburgers. Rather, cholesterol is something our bodies naturally produce. It has a function and a role in our bodies' natural balance and maintenance. It is as normal a part of the human body as enzymes, hormones and blood cells. Without cholesterol we would die.

So, if it is so important, what does cholesterol do?

- Cholesterol is the building block for the sex hormones estrogen and testosterone and for adrenal hormones that help regulate blood pressure and assist us in times of stress.
- It is the main component of bile acids, which aid in digestion. Cholesterol enables us to digest fats and vitamins A, D, E and K.
- It coats the nerves and makes nerve transmission possible.
- It assists in the normal growth of cells, since cells and their contents are rich in cholesterol.
- It gives skin the ability to shed water.
- It protects us from kidney disease in case of diabetes.
- It is important for the growth and repair of brain cells.
- It helps transport blood fats through the circulatory system.[3]

When cholesterol levels are too low, your body is dying, not becoming healthier. Some types of cancer are associated with low cholesterol levels.[4]

FROM WHERE DOES IT COME?

Where does cholesterol come from? More than 80 percent of it is produced by our bodies, and most of that by the liver, though each cell is capable of producing its own cholesterol. In fact, only 7 percent of all the cholesterol in our bodies is in our blood. The rest resides in every cell where it protects and gives structure to cell membranes and regulates the outflow of wastes and inflow of nutrients.[5]

Your body needs large amounts of cholesterol to function, and it works hard to regulate the level of cholesterol. When you eat less cholesterol, your body makes more. When you consume more cholesterol, your body makes less. That is why cholesterol levels have proven stubbornly resistant to efforts to lower them through diet. Tests have repeatedly shown that changing your diet can only alter your cholesterol level 4 percent at the most.[6] But how much is really too much or too little?

WHY LDL CHOLESTEROL IS BAD

There is a very good reason to call cholesterol good and bad. Unhealthy cholesterol is when the level of low-density lipoproteins, or LDL, is too high. This causes dangerous reactions that harm the inside layer of the arteries with inflammation. Such reactions include free-radical activity (a kind of cellular warfare caused by oxidation), the buildup of fatty plaques and platelet adhesion, the process that allows the kind of thickening and stickiness of the blood that you find when a clot forms or when a wound heals. All of these things are recipes for disastrous

61

blood clots, which is why LDL cholesterol is called "bad."

THE PROTECTIVE ROLE
OF HDL CHOLESTEROL

High-density lipoproteins (HDL) help protect your blood vessels against cardiovascular disease. When low-density lipoproteins do their damage, high-density lipoproteins come to the rescue. Here's how they help:

- HDL reverses cholesterol transport, which means it helps remove the bad cholesterol from blood cells, reducing the amount of LDL that gets into the blood vessel walls.
- HDL reduces free-radical activity caused by LDL oxidation.
- HDL restores prostacyclin synthesis.

In other words, HDL is a wonderful multipurpose substance that protects against and reverses the thickening or buildup in the arteries caused by atherosclerosis. No only that, but it is also a powerful antioxidant, an anti-inflammatory agent and a blood-thinning agent all rolled into one.

THE TRUTH ABOUT CHOLESTEROL

The medical community generally views cholesterol as follows: The lower the density of the lipoprotein (LDL), the more harmful the cholesterol is to our health.

Nevertheless, I'd like to challenge this popular notion. You see, I find this thinking difficult to accept. For how can our bodies, within the design of normal function, produce substances that are harmful?

One of the many wonders of the human body is the economy of its function. There are no wasted steps or unnecessary processes. No matter how ugly triglycerides may look to a chemist in the laboratory, they are beautifully necessary to the body. What makes these substances harmful is their excess, but not having enough is just as dangerous. As long as there is a good balance, the system is happy.

A healthy balance of good and bad cholesterol depends on their ratio more than the quantity. The measuring stick for cardiovascular disease risk is as follows:

- Total cholesterol/HDL = <4
- LDL/HDL = <3

Before you panic at a cholesterol count of 280 in your latest blood test, look at your HDL and LDL results. Use these formulas to calculate your ratios; it is a better measure of risk.

Independently of how high or low your "cholesterol" is, if your ratios are within these numbers, your risk of suffering from heart disease is low. Conversely, no matter how low your total cholesterol is, if the ratios of LDL and HDL are higher than these two numbers, your risk of heart disease is much higher. Many factors, such as eating too much saturated fat, can throw this important balance out of whack and increase your risk of heart disease.

NO "CORRECT" LEVEL

Plenty of evidence has always existed that suggests that no particular level of cholesterol is "right." Instead, there is a cholesterol level that is right for you.

This fact was proven in 1998 by a team of scientists from the

University of Texas Southwestern Medical Center and the National Institutes of Health when they discovered a gene responsible for abnormal cholesterol absorption in some people with a rare hereditary disease. Before this discovery, scientists understood very little about how cholesterol is absorbed from what we eat and how it is passed from our bodies.

> "Only a fraction of the cholesterol we consume is actually absorbed by the body," said Dr. Shailendra Patel, assistant professor of clinical nutrition and a scholar in the Center for Human Nutrition at UT Southwestern. "Different people absorb different amounts. Some might eat a cholesterol-laden meal and absorb 30 percent of it; someone else might eat a low-cholesterol meal but absorb 60 percent of it."[7]

UNCERTAIN TEST RESULTS?

Laboratory equipment can make it difficult to measure cholesterol levels accurately. Cholesterol tests are done on the blood, but as I stated earlier, only 7 percent of the body's cholesterol is found in the blood. The rest is dispersed throughout the body.

To demonstrate this, a *Wall Street Journal* reporter sent blood samples to five different labs in New York and got back results that placed him in the high, borderline and low cholesterol categories.[8]

The standards that define "high," "borderline-high" and "desirable" cholesterol levels have been subject to discussion and changes. The levels called "borderline-high" were what should have been called "average," but the idea behind defining cholesterol levels was to inject a measure of fear, and terminology played an important role in conveying that fear.[9]

These inconsistencies cause confusion and overtreatment. A large group of Tennesseans was tested for cholesterol, and 75 percent were found to need medical treatment. However, an additional independent test revealed that only 25 percent should have fallen into treatment categories.[10]

I would dare ask, Was there *really* anybody in need of treatment?

Startling, isn't it? How can I support such an indictment? Let me explain it this way. Much of what we get patients to do is coercive: "If you do not take your medicine, you will surely die." In order for us to be assertive, an illness has to be diagnosed. This is a potential market for the pharmaceutical industry, especially when there is a treatment available. The market potential is directly related to the length of treatment. Establishing cholesterol "standards" converts an impressive number of perfectly asymptometic people with extremely doubtful potential risk into patients. Since this is a condition that is not curable, these "patients" will have to take the *proper* treatment for life. A pretty good formula for success I would dare say.

> HDL is a wonderful multipurpose substance that protects against and reverses the thickening or buildup in the arteries caused by athero-sclerosis.

HOW BAD IS CHOLESTEROL?

Eating high levels of dietary cholesterol may not make as much of a difference as we have been led to believe. Consuming dietary cholesterol raises overall cholesterol as well as increasing LDL cholesterol levels. As we know, elevated levels are associated with an increased risk of heart disease.

However, most studies show that dietary cholesterol has less effect upon blood cholesterol than dietary fatty acids. Nevertheless, dietary cholesterol may act synergistically with these fatty acids. Saturated fatty acids dramatically increase overall and LDL cholesterol levels.

SHOULD CHOLESTEROL BE RESTRICTED?

Although the relationship between dietary cholesterol and blood cholesterol concentrations is complex, it is generally recommended that cholesterol, along with saturated fat, should be restricted in the diet. But should they?

Shepherds in Somalia eat almost nothing but milk from their camels, about a gallon and a half per day, which means they consume about a pound of butter fat per day. But their cholesterol is much lower than in most western countries.[11]

Among Arctic Eskimos, Kenyan Kikuyu and Masai, American Navajos, Australian aborigines and in other cultures that eat traditional, primitive diets, no signs of arteriosclerosis or heart disease are found, even in the very old. They have never been worried about their *good, bad* and *ugly* cholesterols. (Several researchers, nevertheless, have found that the average total cholesterol levels in these societies is around 150 instead of the 200 level accepted in the medical world.) However, when they search for financial health through the

"American Dream" in Western cultures or become affluent in their own countries, they start eating *light* and *healthy* processed nonfoods and surprisingly begin to get *heavy* and *sick* independently of their blood cholesterol level.

U.S. studies confirm this. One of the authors of the Framingham study wrote that variations in blood cholesterol levels were in no way connected to diet.[12] A study in Michigan found that those with low blood cholesterol ate just as much saturated fat as those with high cholesterol.[13]

> Eating high levels of dietary cholesterol may not make as much of a difference as we have been led to believe.

In fact, no evidence exists that too much cholesterol in the diet promotes heart attacks or hardening of the arteries. If a high cholesterol level hardened the arteries, then people with high cholesterol should have more atherosclerosis, but that is simply not so.[14] Diet does little or nothing to change our cholesterol level. Even if it did, there is no study showing that cholesterol causes heart attacks.

Author Artemis Simopoulos, M.D., argues that if all adults were to go on cholesterol-lowering diets for the rest of their lives, life expectancy in the U.S. would increase by only three months for women and four months for men.[15]

CHOLESTEROL DRUGS

A number of clinical trials have reported that cholesterol-lowering drugs are more effective in reducing blood cholesterol levels. Is that true? Cautiously speaking, yes.

Four clinical trials undertaken with four different drugs (Atromid, Lopid, Questran and Lestid) were very effective in bringing down cholesterol levels. Nevertheless, the "drugged" group of people who were tested had the same or an even lower survival rate than those who didn't receive drugs. In other words, the patients with high cholesterol and no drugs fared better than the patients with lower cholesterol!

> No evidence exists that too much cholesterol in the diet promotes heart attacks or hardening of the arteries.

Unbelievably, in one of the studies, the group receiving a placebo had an almost 30 percent better survival rate!

In a notorious study conducted in Finland in 1987, called the Helsinki Heart Study, another cholesterol-lowering drug called gemfibrozil was given to more than four thousand patients. The drug lowered cholesterol and heart attacks—but here again the control group realized a better overall survival rate.[16]

Cholesterol-lowering drugs like Zocor and Pravachol have been shown to decrease the incidence of death due to heart disease and stroke, but some question remains as to what is causing the improvement. For instance, because of these results cardiologists are now recommending "cholesterol-lowering" treatment to patients with angina or with a history of heart attack, but with *normal* cholesterol levels, suggesting that lowering cholesterol may not be the reason these drugs work.[17]

And while the drugs save lives, many of them are prescribed

for people who would not experience a heart attack anyway. In other words, the drugs are taken preventively by thousands, but save the lives of just a few. Is it worth the possible side effects, especially that of increasing the risk of cancer, to make such drugs widely available and to advertise them heavily in magazines and on television, giving people the impression that their fears can be allayed at no other cost to their health?

You may say, "Yeah, it's worth the risk." But since deciding who *really* is at risk is blurry at best, most of the people taking the cholesterol-lowering drugs are basically just exposed to the side effects. It's like throwing a bomb with someone's name on it into a crowded restaurant.

THE REAL CULPRIT

It is possible that we were better off when we knew nothing about cholesterol! Now we eat low-cholesterol foods and think we're helping our hearts. Or we have created stress-related problems by worrying excessively about our cholesterol levels! I'm being facetious, of course. But the fact remains that cholesterol alone plays a minor role in the development of heart disease.

The problem is not the cholesterol but the rest of the diet. Cholesterol may be an indicator of poor lifestyle choices, but it is not the culprit itself. It is an independent variable. Cholesterol levels have remained constant for decades while heart disease has risen and declined.[18] In the words of one researcher, "There is no increase in overall mortality with either high or low cholesterol."[19]

In America, arteriosclerosis—that arterial sludge that acts so much like the dirty sediment at the mouth of the muddy Mississippi River—begins in childhood. It is the buildup of plaque in the arteries caused by many factors—factors that we have ignored. Prevention and treatment of dangerous levels of cholesterol have not yielded the expected results, and angioplasty and heart bypasses are designed to just bridge but not to cure the problem.

If you are still worried about your high cholesterol count, there are much more effective ways to lower it than cholesterol-lowering drugs. Diet and exercise, the subject of the next chapters, are the most powerful keys that will help you prevent and even reverse arteriosclerosis. Let's look.

Chapter 5

Are You
Eating Heart Smart?

Have you ever rushed into a convenience store when stopping for gas and scanned the aisles for something to eat to tide you over until you found time for a meal? You found row upon row of expensive, shiny packages filled with processed fatty and sugary items of various shapes, sizes and often amazingly unnatural colors, rows of chocolate bars, cookies, gooey pastries, orange and pink powdery chips and bright-blue flavored drinks.

No, this won't do, you think to yourself. You need real food. So, running to the refrigerated section you scan the misty rows for nourishment. There's processed meat probably made with 20 percent animal hair. Ugh. No! White bread that will wrap around your incisors like Super glue. Nah!

You go to the counter looking for a simple piece of fruit. A hard, dark red apple looks too perfect and could last in a fruit dish for several months, if not longer.

So many eating choices, but very little food. Whether you eat something or leave hungry, the result will be the same—

you will be left unsatisfied. You check your watch and shake your head as the glass doors close behind you.

What has happened to us?

What you eat is one of your most significant keys for preventing and reversing heart disease.

Food sustains us, and it can be a source of considerable pleasure. It is a reflection of our rich social fabric and cultural heritage. It brings families together and becomes part of our fondest memories. And so it is that when anyone attempts to infringe on this most coveted of pleasures, resistance is inevitable. We seem to think it is our right to eat whatever we want, whenever we want, without consequences.

> Hippocrates said that you enjoy health only if you and your body are in perfect balance with the environment.

Few would argue that changing our diets could vastly improve our health and reduce a great deal of needless suffering on a worldwide level. Improving our diet appears to be a universally accepted goal, but our good intentions have become obscured. At the center of the confusion are cholesterol and fat intake—important factors in beating heart disease, no doubt, but certainly no culprits.

Political and economical interests have muddied the waters even more. Their efforts to educate us against dietary evils have not caused us to eat healthier. Instead, we have created policies and methods of handling foods that have not improved our health. Industries offer health through empty calories, fake fats, non-calorie sweeteners and the like. Such wonders have given us little more than false confidence. They haven't nourished our bodies. Instead, they have created a false confidence that we are getting healthier when the opposite is true.

On one hand the government's attempts to educate people about food is commendable. But on the other hand, the government's policy to protect industry's nonfood is appalling. Extreme chemical (and other) manipulation of foodstuffs to increase productivity, shelf life and economical gain contribute to the very explosion of the diseases it has targeted to prevent, diseases such as heart disease, cancer and diabetes.

Confusion reigns in the field of natural approaches to health. Orthodox and unorthodox health professionals (and nonprofessionals) strongly disagree and probably will never come to terms of agreement. Natural food supplies are quite varied, and possibilities for management and prevention are as diverse.

The American Heart Association continues to recommend a high carbohydrate/low-fat diet. But increasingly doctors are telling their patients to reconsider.

According to Dr. Michael Eades, "Many researchers are already on board the movement away from processed grains and sugar. Many physicians are also quickly moving in this direction. At this point, organizations like the American Diabetes Association are trying to save face by *slowly* changing their focus away from a high-carbohydrate diet. It would be embarrassing to do a 180-degree turn and admit that they haven't been right all of these years."[1]

NUTRITIONAL BALANCE

Hippocrates said that you enjoy health only if you and your

body are in perfect balance with the environment. Eating habits have become severely unbalanced in the past one hundred to two hundred years. Fat consumption has increased dramatically from about 20 percent of the energy intake in the middle of the nineteenth century to about 50 percent today, despite the fact that people today need much less energy because they are far less physically active.[2]

People have taken to eating high-calorie foods at the expense of low-calorie foods like plant starches and fibers, which during the same period have been reduced to one-half of the amount people used to eat. People are not consuming nearly as many vitamins, phyto-nutrients, antioxidants and other important substances found in fresh fruits, vegetables, nuts and whole grains.

> The food that the Bible recommends, and the general principles we find in its pages, can keep our hearts healthier than any diet on the market today.

One person consumes approximately sixty tons of food in his or her lifetime, comparable to five to ten tractor-trailers full. Have you ever thought about what your load looks like? Is it piled high with candy and potato chips? Does it look like you won the M&M sweepstakes? Or is it full of leafy green foods and a good balance of fruits, breads, meats, milks and so on?

There are many diets in the popular culture today. Some doctors promote high-protein diets. Some say carbohydrates are the cure. Some people have used evidence that vegetarians have very low rates of heart disease to promote vegetarian diets, but the popular concept that vegetarianism is the healthiest lifestyle has been under attack and scientific evidence is mounting against it. High-profile doctors like Robert Atkins (a proponent of bacon and eggs) and Dean Ornish (broccoli and so forth) will put their lives on the line to defend their theories for a universal diet, based, they say, on irrefutable scientific evidence.

Whose expert advice should we follow? Sparks were flying between Dean Ornish and Atkins in a heated debate over carbohydrate vs. protein diet at a conference I attended in Orlando not too long ago. Both best-selling authors regaled each other with evidence and testimonials.

I am sure their debate won over some, confused many and entertained all. But I am afraid that, in the end, they only fanned the flames of confusion. What we desperately need is practical, unbiased, unrestricted, non-discriminative, universal dietary wisdom.

But where can we find such good-for-all diet? After so much has been searched and researched, am I going to propose an even newer diet? No, I am not. The advice I want to give in the next two chapters may seem new to many, but it actually is very old.

THE GOOD BOOK

The universal dietary "laws" I propose are found in the Bible, the oldest record of lifestyle recommendations in history. The food that the Bible recommends, and the general principles we find in its pages, can keep our hearts healthier than any diet on the market today.

The Bible was astonishingly ahead of its time. Indeed, the

dietary recommendations in Exodus, Leviticus, Numbers and Deuteronomy have been called "a bold leap into the future, a giant stride ahead of anything existing at that time." It was not until five hundred years later that the Sumerian code was augmented and incorporated by the Babylonians into the Code of Hammurabi, but these laws did not have the democratic spirit of the Torah.

We know of no written Roman laws until the second century B.C. The concept that we are all equal before the law, a law based on a written code, comes from the Semitic people. The Sumerians, whose written code of laws dates back to 2500 B.C., were probably the first people on earth to have a written law, but it lacked the sense of justice that Mosaic Law contained. But the Jewish precepts, in contrast with all others, were not limited to social behavior; the Mosaic code is quite singular because it also includes strict lifestyle and dietary measures auguring benefits and consequences depending on whether you adopt or reject the recommendations.

The Jewish dietary laws came in the context of the entire Mosaic Law. These laws are a prescription for healthy living whether you are Jew or Chinese, Christian or Buddist, believer or atheist. This code obviously is soaked in spiritual undertones, but if you want to remove all the cultural and religious nuances, the health and preventive wisdom is, in spite of being more than four thousand years old, very much up-to-date. Nevertheless, in keeping with the rules of editing, as I have respected the researchers' authorship and have quoted them verbatim, I will do so with the biblical references.

Deuteronomy 14:3 states, "Do not eat any detestable thing" (NIV). Imagine if Moses had known about hot dogs, which contain more detestable things than you can imagine, including up to 20 percent animal hair!

Moses said:

> So the LORD commanded us to observe all these statutes, to fear the LORD our God for our good always and for our survival, as it is today.
>
> —DEUTERONOMY 6:24, NAS

God wanted a people who were healthy, not afflicted by illness, so He gave them laws of various types, telling them how to eat, work, have sexual relations and so on. God's laws were very specific. For example, He forbade them from drinking blood, which we now know carries all sorts of diseases and can make a person very sick.

The point was to have a people who thrived spiritually and physically, who lived long and prosperous lives. The Law promised health. It said:

> The LORD will remove from you all sickness; and He will not put on you any of the harmful diseases of Egypt which you have known.
>
> —DEUTERONOMY 7:15, NAS

Interestingly, in studying hundreds of Egyptian mummies, paleontologists have discovered recently that these people were affected by arteriosclerosis, diabetes, cancer, arthritis and many of the disease that plague our world today. Their health was precarious due to their unhealthy lifestyles, especially their eating habits. In other words, they ate contrary to biblical health wisdom.[3]

So the Jews, in order to stay healthy, had to follow the

prescription. These laws proclaimed the responsibility of personal choices:

> Biblical prevention wisdom is universal, and if you follow it, you will drastically reduce your chances of heart disease.

I call heaven and earth as witnesses today against you, that I have set before you life and death, blessing and cursing; therefore choose life, that both you and your descendants may live.

—DEUTERONOMY 30:19

"Choose life." How those words ring today through our grocery stores and fast-food restaurants! Yet who heeds them? Who is choosing life with their diet? For those who found it "too difficult," the Law promised curses of all kinds.

If you are not careful to observe all the words of this law which are written in this book, to fear this honored and awesome name, the LORD your God, then the LORD will bring extraordinary plagues on you and your descendants, even severe and lasting plagues, and miserable and chronic sicknesses. And He will bring back on you all the diseases of Egypt of which you were afraid, and they shall cling to you. Also every sickness and every plague which, not written in the book of this law, the LORD will bring on you until you are destroyed. Then you shall be left few in number, whereas you were as the stars of heaven for multitude, because you did not obey the LORD your God.

—DEUTERONOMY 28:58–62, NAS

Elsewhere in the Bible, the Lord spoke through the prophet Hosea, saying, "My people are destroyed for lack of knowledge" (Hos. 4:6). This means knowledge of all kinds, including health.

The apostle John wrote, "Beloved, I wish above all things that thou mayest prosper and be in health, even as thy soul prospereth" (3 John 2, KJV).

Throughout the Bible God refers to health as part of His package of blessings given to obedient people. He would not promise health without giving us keys to having it. Those keys are found in the specific dietary laws in the Bible and in the general principles we can observe.

The biblical prevention wisdom that we are about to explore is, after more than four thousand years, up-to-date and validated by modern scientific methodology. These laws apply to you whether you prefer vegetarianism or omnivorism; whether your emotional type matches your blood type; whether you are brown or yellow, young or old, female or male, believer or not. Biblical prevention wisdom is universal, and if you follow it, you will drastically reduce your chances of heart disease.

FOOD AFFECTS THE HEART

Believe it or not, though the Bible has long linked the diet to health, many modern people rejected the idea that the diet caused heart disease until very recently. It took skeptical scientists and doctors decades to "decide" that diet could cause or prevent disease. A major statement was made in 1989 when Surgeon General C. Everett Koop issued a report on nutrition and health. In the preface, the assistant secretary for health wrote:

> **The foods we eat are the most important single factor in determining whether or not we develop heart disease.**

Diseases such as coronary heart disease, stroke, cancer and diabetes remain leading causes of death and disability in the United States. Substantial scientific research over the past few decades indicates that diet can play an important role in prevention of such conditions.[4]

The report said firmly that heart disease was linked to excessive or unbalanced diets and that a reduction in the intake of fat and other foods should reduce the risk of heart disease.[5]

This report ends any scientific controversy. There is no doubt that diet affects chronic-disease risk. In addition, because of the enormity of the impact of diet-related diseases, the report demonstrates that virtually all Americans will benefit from following these recommendations.

Even though the results of various individual studies may be inconclusive, the preponderance of the evidence presented in the report's comprehensive scientific review substantiates an association between dietary factors and rates of chronic diseases.[6]

Of course, the Bible would have ended the "controversy" years ago, but who looks to the Bible for dinner recommendations these days? Not many. And yet it is the template for a healthy diet.

The foods we eat are the most important single factor in determining whether or not we develop heart disease. Let's look at the heart-healthy foods we want in our pantries and refrigerators, based on what the Bible recommends.

FRUITS AND VEGETABLES

The very best thing you can do for your heart from a dietary point of view is to eat more fruits and vegetables. They are the backbone of any heart-healthy diet.

Biblical wisdom reflects this fact. It says:

> Then God said, "I give you every seed-bearing plant on the face of the whole earth and every tree that has fruit with seed in it. They will be yours for food."
>
> —GENESIS 1:29, NIV

The Bible tells us that God intended that we eat vegetables to maintain our health. It says:

> He causes the grass to grow for the cattle, and vegetation for the service of man.
>
> —PSALM 104:14

And again:

> The bread and summer fruit [are] for the young men to eat.
>
> —2 SAMUEL 16:2

81

Modern science backs up what the biblical laws told us thousands of years ago. Studies show time and again that people who eat a lot of fruits and vegetables have reduced risk of heart disease.[7] In Finland during the early 1970s, people began eating substantially more fruit and vegetables. This change correlated directly with a decline in death from heart disease.[8]

Dr. Dean Ornish at the University of California, San Francisco, found that people in his study who ate vegetarian diets that were low in fat had half the number of heart problems as people who ate the typical American diet. Not just that, but they lost thirteen pounds and kept it off for four years![9]

Fruits and vegetables don't contain cholesterol, and they are naturally low in fat, saturated fat, calories and sodium. They are also rich in protein, potassium, fiber, folic acid and vitamin C.

A study in Italy showed that high vegetable consumption decreased heart attacks by 21 percent and chest pain by 11 percent.[10] A diet high in fruits and vegetables, including nuts, actually lowers blood pressure.[11]

Fruits and vegetables are also rich in phytochemicals, biologically active plant compounds that are "semi-essential" but are not classified currently as vitamins or minerals. There are three classes of phytochemicals that help prevent heart disease. They are:

- Plant sterols
- Flavonoids
- Plant sulfur compounds

Sterols appear to block cholesterol absorption from the diet or increase cholesterol excretion from the body.[12]

Flavonoids extend the activity of vitamin C, act as free-radical scavengers, prevent LDL cholesterol oxidation (delaying the development of hard arteries), inhibit platelet aggregation and have anti-inflammatory action.[13]

Flavonoid intake has been shown to reduce the fatality of heart disease and the incidence of heart attack. In the Zutphen Elderly Study, elderly men with the highest consumption of flavonoids over a five-year period had 60 percent less mortality from heart disease than low flavonoid consumers.[14]

> If you love your heart, you will decide right now to add more fruits and vegetables to your diet.

Women are dramatically helped, too. A study of post-menopausal women found a 38 percent reduction in heart disease deaths in the highest category of total flavonoid intake compared with the lowest. In this study, broccoli was shown to have a statistically significant effect on reducing heart disease.[15]

Plant sulfur compounds are found in the allium family of vegetables, which includes garlic, onions and leeks. It has been shown that garlic possesses preventive and protective properties against cardiovascular disease.[16]

Pigments provide color to fruits and vegetables, and they also protect us from heart disease. *Anthocyanins* are the water-soluble, reddish pigments found in many fruits, such as strawberries, cherries, raspberries, cranberries, blueberries, grapes and black currants. Anthocyanins in fruits provide protection against heart disease by slowing the generation of cholesterol.[17]

Carotenoids are the pigments found in yellow-orange, red and green vegetables and yellow-orange fruits. The carotenoids are powerful antioxidants that quench free radicals, protect against oxidative damage and help our immune system.[18]

Eating veggies even helps our bodies maintain a balance of blood sugar. A study conducted in Britain found that people who ate salad and raw vegetables frequently year-round had an over 80 percent lower risk of adult-onset diabetes than people who ate vegetables less often.

"FIVE A DAY"

Eating five servings of fruits and vegetables every day can make all the difference for your heart health. Unfortunately, the average American eats fewer than two servings of vegetables per day and less than one serving of fruit. A nationwide campaign called "Five a Day for Better Health" encourages people to eat at least five servings a day of fruit and vegetables.

If you love your heart, you will decide right now to add more fruits and vegetables to your diet. If you already eat plenty of them, I applaud you. If not, make it a habit. Buy apples instead of potato chips, oranges instead of candy bars, and stock your fridge and fruit bowl with bananas, kiwi fruit and whatever else is in season. Availability makes all the difference in the world.

After just a few days or weeks your body will begin to crave these foods as you used to crave unhealthy foods.

I promise you, your heart will leap for joy!

OLIVE OIL

Olive oil is another food mentioned often in the Bible for its many healthful attributes. The Bible tells us that olive oil will strengthen our hearts, and scientific facts prove that this is so.

Psalm 104:14−15 says:

> He causes the grass to grow for the cattle, and vegetation for the service of man, that he may bring forth food from the earth, and wine that makes glad the heart of man, oil to make his face shine, and bread which strengthens man's heart.

Deuteronomy 8:7−8 tells us that olive oil is a part of the best that God has given us.

> For the LORD your God is bringing you into a good land...a land of olive oil and honey.

Olive oil is one of the healthiest oils on the planet. Perhaps it is because plants in the Mediterranean experience long exposure to sunlight, increasing the levels of flavonoids, anthocyanins and phenols in the olives.

The phenols in olive oil are antioxidants, inhibiting oxidation of low-density lipoprotein (LDL) and getting rid of free radicals. When we eat olive oil, our arteries experience less damage.[19]

Italian scientists recently reported that patients with high blood pressure reduced the amount of drugs they needed to lower their blood pressure by switching to a diet low in

> Olive oil is a wonderful cooking aid and works well as a substitute for butter or margarine.

saturated fat and rich in olive oil. What's more, some of the patients were able to stop their high blood pressure medication completely with the dietary changes.

A slight reduction in saturated fat intake, along with the use of extra-virgin olive oil, markedly lowers the need for high blood pressure drugs. Similar results were not found in people who ate more sunflower oil. Olive oil was able to reduce the need for blood pressure medication because it contains polyphenols, which are antioxidant compounds that may help to open arteries and reduce blood pressure.[20]

Again, the phenols in olive oil are responsible for reducing the need for blood pressure medication because they increase the production of substances that help open arteries, which in turn reduces artery resistance to the blood flow, and blood pressure is decreased.

Olive oil is a wonderful cooking aid and works well as a substitute for butter or margarine. Instead of putting a stick of butter on the table, put in a small bowl some virgin olive oil, a bit of vinegar and a spinkle of herbs. You and your family will enjoy the taste, and your heart will be healthier.

NUTS

Nuts are also mentioned in the Bible for their health benefits. Let's look.

Genesis 43:11 says, "And their father Israel said unto them, If it must be so now, do this; take of the best fruits in the land in your vessels, and carry down the man a present, a little balm, and a little honey, spices, and myrrh, nuts, and almonds" (KJV).

Traditionally, nuts have been off limits to people on diets because of their high fat content. Indeed, about 60 percent of the weight and 80 percent of the calories in most nuts come from fat. But five of the best and largest studies report that eating nuts frequently is associated with a decreased risk of heart disease. In fact, no other food has been so consistently associated with a marked reduction in heart disease risk in people of all habits, races and health profiles.[21]

Those who eat lots of nuts experience an extra 5.6 years of life expectancy free of heart disease and an 18 percent lifetime risk of heart disease compared with 30 percent in people who eat few nuts.[22] A 50-gram serving of nuts exceeds the recommended daily allowance for vitamin E, which has been shown to reduce the risk of coronary heart disease.[23]

You would do well to incorporate nuts into your daily life, whether that means including them in your recipes or keeping a bowl of them on the table. For the health-conscious person, nuts are no longer taboo.

GRAPE JUICE

Grapes are one of the most widely consumed fruits in the world, and they have wonderfully heart-healthy attributes. Deuteronomy 23:24 says, "When you come into your neighbor's vineyard, you may eat your fill of grapes."

In a very recent study, drinking an average of about two cups (450 ml.) of purple grape juice a day for one week vastly reduced the "stickiness" of blood platelets. By comparison, orange juice and grapefruit juice showed no effect on platelet aggregation. The difference may be due to the different kinds of flavonoids they contain. Purple grape juice also has approximately three times the total polyphenolic concentration of citrus juices. Polyphenols are powerful antioxidants.[24]

In another study platelets were incubated in a grape juice

dilution, which, it was shown, helped to make the platelets less sticky. Grape juice also appears to contribute to increasing the opening of the arteries. Then the platelet inhibitory effect of grape juice decreases the risk of coronary thrombosis (clots) and heart attack.[25]

Eating our fill of grapes would do most of us a world of good. Every child who has toted their lunch to school in a brown paper bag knows how good a cluster of grapes can taste in the middle of the day. Crisp and refreshing, they burst with flavor and life.

Take a bunch of grapes to work instead of waiting for the afternoon break to buy a candy bar from the vending machine. You may be taking a "blood thinner" precribed by your doctor to prevent a heart attack, which is not a bad idea (the most common one is Coumadin). But in case you didn't know, it's exactly what the exterminators use to poison rats! If you take this advice, you may lower the amount of Coumadin, or if your doctor determines that your blood is thin enough, you may even do without it! This ancient wisdom can become a delicious snack—and may help to save your life.

Consider replacing soda and sugary-sweet drinks with refreshing grape juice. Again, availability of this healthy drink in your refrigerator will make the difference.

ALCOHOL

In the 1990s, a remarkably consistent body of evidence was collected suggesting that those who drink alcohol moderately have a reduced risk of coronary heart disease compared to abstainers. This preventive effect of alcohol may be largely confined to middle-aged and older subjects.[26]

In contrast, binge drinking, particularly by young men, and chronic heavy drinking can negate the heart-healthy benefits of alcohol. Instead, such patterns of drinking increase the risk of hypertension, hemorrhagic and ischemic stroke and heart disease and heart attacks.[27]

The relation between alcohol and risk of heart disease has been described as a J-shaped curve, in which the equivalent of two drinks per day of any kind of alcohol is associated with a 50 percent reduction risk compared with nondrinkers. At the same time, higher doses, such as six drinks per day, increase the risk of heart attack and stroke twofold. These observations show that light drinking protects against death, heart attack or hospitalization for heart disease in every one of the diverse populations studied and in both sexes.[28]

> In the 1990s, a remarkably consistent body of evidence was collected suggesting that those who drink alcohol moderately have a reduced risk of coronary heart disease compared to abstainers.

There are many theories about why alcohol reduces heart disease. At least half of the protective action appears to be explained by an increase in HDL ("good") cholesterol. Alcohol also keeps blood platelets from sticking and piling up on artery walls.

All of this poses a dilemma from a public health and a religious standpoint. How do people who are morally opposed to drinking alcohol incorporate this knowledge into their lifestyles, or do they? The best way is to consult your own conscience. The benefits of drinking alcohol are not significant enough to go against one's morals, and most of the beneficial effects of alcohol can be achieved by a low-fat diet alone. But the heart does seem to benefit from moderate alcohol consumption.

> Red wine might help explain the "French paradox": the fact that the incidence of heart disease mortality in France is the lowest among industrial countries despite the high incidence of risk factors such as smoking, a high-fat diet and lack of exercise.

RED WINE

The most heart-healthy alcoholic drink is red wine, which contains abundant polyphenols that have a wonderful effect on our cardiovascular system. (White wine does not have nearly the same positive impact.) Red wine has been shown to inhibit LDL cholesterol oxidation, help prevent atherosclerosis, increase antioxidant capacity and raise plasma levels of HDL ("good") cholesterol.[29]

Wisdom from the Bible supports this, too. Deuteronomy 33:28 says, "Then Israel shall dwell in safety, the fountain of Jacob alone, in a land of grain and new wine; his heavens shall also drop dew."

And again in 1 Chronicles 16:2–3, the Bible says, "And

when David had made an end of offering the burnt offerings and the peace offerings, he blessed the people in the name of the LORD. And he dealt to every one of Israel, both man and woman, to every one a loaf of bread, and a good piece of flesh, and a flagon of wine" (KJV).

Red wine might help explain the "French paradox": the fact that the incidence of heart disease mortality in France is the lowest among industrial countries despite the high incidence of risk factors such as smoking, a high-fat diet and lack of exercise among French people.[30]

Drinking two servings (240–280 ml.) of red wine per day will provide approximately 40 percent of the total antioxidant polyphenols present in a healthy diet, as well as polyphenols like resveratrol that are virtually absent from fruit and vegetables. Wine holds an advantage over vegetables in that its polyphenols are much more available for our body's use. Only tea can approach the advantages of wine in this respect.

TEA

Aside from water, tea is the most widely consumed drink in the world. It is also heart healthy. Thirty-five to 50 percent of extractable solids of green tea leaves are polyphenolic compounds. A single cup of green tea usually contains about 200–400 milligrams of polyphenols. Green tea shows stronger antioxidant activity than the black tea more common in America.

Studies have indicated that drinking tea protects against heart disease.[31]

COFFEE

For almost seventy years it has been recognized that moderate doses of caffeine elevate blood pressure. Coffee has been associated with an increased risk of stroke in men over the age of fifty-five with high blood pressure. The risk was more than doubled for men who consumed three cups of coffee per day compared to people who did not drink coffee.[32]

Despite the general impression that high coffee consumption is bad, the Scottish Heart Study found the prevalence of heart disease to be the highest among those who abstain from coffee drinking and lowest among those who drink five or more cups per day in Scotland.[33]

Whatever your coffee habits are, some restriction of regular coffee intake may be beneficial in older individuals with high blood pressure.

CHOCOLATE

Recently it was shown that chocolate contains large amounts of flavonoid polyphenols that have potent antioxidant activities.[34] Forty-one grams of milk chocolate contain almost as many polyphenols as a standard serving of red wine.[35]

The flavonoid polyphenols in chocolate help to prevent hardening of the arteries. Research suggests that dietary intake of chocolate may reduce the risk of atherosclerosis and morbidity and mortality from heart disease.

Of course, eating too much chocolate is not recommended. Chocolate is made with large amounts of refined sugar. But if you want an occasional sugary snack, chocolate is a good alternative.

FATS

The Bible warns against eating fat. Leviticus 7:23 says, "You shall not eat any fat, of ox or sheep or goat."

Fat is a major culprit in the development of heart disease, but it depends on the kind of fat and how much is consumed. Animal fats are among the worst for our hearts. Recent findings from the Oxford Vegetarian Study show that vegetarians and vegans had a 39 percent lower death rate due to heart disease than people who eat meat at least once a week. Fish eaters showed similar results as vegetarians. There is a strong correlation between higher consumption of animal fats and the risk of death by heart disease.[36]

It appears that animal fats are harmful, but other fats are not, if eaten in moderation. The highest coronary heart disease mortality rates in the world are in Eastern bloc countries in which lard and beef tallow are cornerstones of the diet.[37]

Other fats, like those from olive and canola oils, are healthier. Recent studies have shown that monounsaturated fatty acids, like those in olive and canola oils, bring down plasma cholesterol levels.[38]

About 50 percent of saturated fat and 70 percent of cholesterol in the U.S. diet come from hamburgers, cheeseburgers, meat loaf, whole milk, cheese, other dairy products (including ice cream), beef steaks, roasts, hot dogs, ham, lunch meat, doughnuts, cookies, cakes and eggs.

To reduce the risk of coronary heart disease, people should restrict these foods and eat poultry (white meat without the skin), fish, nonfat or low-fat yogurt, low-fat cheeses and drink

> Fat is a major culprit in the development of heart disease, but it depends on the kind of fat and how much is consumed.

skim or low-fat milk. Unsaturated vegetable oils such as soybean, corn, olive and canola are also good, but they should be eaten in moderation because they are high in calories. Consumption of foods rich in hydrogenated vegetable oils (stick margarine, cookies and French fries) should be avoided.

But let's not fall into the trap of excluding all fat from our diet. God specifically calls fatty foods like butter and curds blessings. (See Deuteronomy 32:14; Isaiah 7:15.) It appears that butter, long labeled an enemy of health by dieticians, is healthier than margarine.[39]

The key is moderation and eating the right kinds of fat—not animal fat or non-naturally occurring fats, but the fats found in nuts and healthy oils. If we do this, it will never be said of us…

> Their heart is as fat as grease.
>
> —PSALM 119:70

FIBER

Ancient biblical laws are not silent regarding the health benefits of fiber. Psalm 81:16 says, "He would have fed them also with the finest of wheat."

Over the past twenty years, many studies have investigated the association between dietary fiber and risk for coronary heart disease. The evidence strongly suggests that dietary fiber reduces the risk of heart disease.

Clinical trials have shown that fiber intake reduces the risk of heart disease, and recent studies suggest that the intake of whole grains like wheat, rice and oats has the strongest preventive effect on heart disease.[40]

Results from the Adventist Health Study revealed that those who ate whole-wheat bread, what the Bible might consider the "finest" of wheat, had fewer heart attacks than those who ate white bread. The risk was far less for people who ate whole-wheat bread than those who ate white bread, which contains very little fiber.[41]

Another study among postmenopausal women showed that those who ate more whole grain experienced 33 percent less risk of heart disease death when compared with people who ate little or no whole grain.[42]

There are two kinds of fiber: soluble fibers, like fruit fibers, which dissolve in water; and nonsoluble fibers, from cereal (meaning grains, not Froot Loops), which do not dissolve in water. Soluble, viscous fibers like psyllium, oat bran, guar and pectin decrease serum cholesterol and LDL cholesterol serum levels, which may contribute to their protective role against heart disease.

> Clinical trials have shown that fiber intake reduces the risk of heart disease.

Cereal fiber has powerful heart-smart benefits, too. From the Nurses' Health Study, it was observed among different sources of dietary fiber (e.g., cereal, vegetables or fruit), that only cereal fiber was strongly associated with a reduced risk of heart disease—19 percent reduction in the risk per 10 grams per day increase in total fiber, and 37 percent reduction in the risk per 5 grams per day increase in cereal fiber. Almost the same results were observed in men in the Health Professionals Follow-up Study. And all these benefits are without the risk of drugs!

Results from the Nurses' Health Study also show that

95

women in the group who ate the most whole grain, which was about 2.5 servings per day, experienced more than 30 percent lower risk of heart disease than the group who ate little whole grain.[43]

Unfortunately, when four thousand American households were surveyed, the results were pitifully unhealthy. The average consumption of whole-grain products is only about 0.5 servings per day per person.[44]

The Food Guide Pyramid of the U.S. Department of Agriculture recommends six to eleven servings of grain products per day, but the amount of whole grains is not specified. Most of the grain products consumed in the U.S. are highly refined, causing them to lose 99 percent of their fiber. The bran (outer layer) and germ (inner layer) are separated from the starchy endosperm (middle layer) during milling.

To get whole-grain products, you only need to look for them. Whole-grain breads, cereals and flour are available in virtually any grocery store, but beware. Look for the grains; some brands are just painted brown. It's about time you had the best part of the grain.

FISH

Biblical laws were very specific about eating fish: "These you may eat of all that are in the water: whatever in the water has fins and scales, whether in the seas or in the rivers—that you may eat" (Lev. 11:9).

Jesus ate fish on several occasions. When He returned from the dead and appeared to the disciples, He asked for fish and ate it in front of them (Luke 24:43). When the crowd was hungry one day, He multiplied fish and bread for them to eat (John 6:1–13). And when Jesus appeared to the disciples on the Sea of Galilee after His resurrection, He cooked fish for them over an open fire (John 21:9).

Fish are a major source of Omega-3 (n-3) fatty acids, which are important to the human body. They help build tissue membranes, especially the retinas and brain. Our body needs them from the day we are conceived.[45]

The n-3 fatty acids from fish and plant sources protect against heart disease and prevent deaths from heart disease and heart attack. The unique properties of n-3 fatty acids in heart disease first became apparent when researchers were studying the health status of Greenland Eskimos who consumed diets very high in fat from seals, whales and fish, and yet had a low rate of heart disease.[46]

Further studies clarified the paradox. The fat Eskimos consumed contained large quantities of the very long chain and highly polyunsaturated fatty acids that are abundant in fish, shellfish and sea mammals, especially in those from cold water, and are scarce or absent in land animals and plants.[47]

Some fatty fish, most notably mackerel, herring, salmon and halibut, are rich sources of n-3 fatty acids.[48]

Plants also provide a rich source of n-3 fatty acids. Vegetable oils like canola, cottonseed and soybean oils are a major source. Coconut, palm and palm kennel oils are not. Other plant sources include nuts, seeds, vegetables, legumes, grains and some fruit. Of these specific foods, nuts, seeds and soybeans are relatively high in n-3 fatty acids.[49]

In recent years, the best level of n-3 fatty acids in the diet has been debated. There have been recommendations that would require fourfold increase in fish consumption in the U.S. or the use of supplements. I tend to agree that most people should eat much more fish than they probably do.

Dietary n-3 fatty acids reduce heart disease risk by preventing fatal cardiac arrhythmias, preventing the formation of blood clots, widening the arteries, inhibiting plaque formation, reducing high blood pressure and preventing arteries from becoming inflamed.[50]

> Fish are a major source of Omega-3 (n-3) fatty acids, which are important to the human body. Our body needs them from the day we are conceived.

In one study, men who ate salmon more than once a week had a 70 percent reduction in the risk of primary cardiac arrest.[51] In another study, total mortality was decreased by 29 percent in men with overt cardiovascular disease who ate n-3 fatty acids from fish or fish oil.[52] In a third study, a diet rich in n-3 fatty acids was given to a group of heart attack survivors, and they experienced a 76 percent decrease in cardiac deaths (secondary prevention) compared with the group of patients that received a conventional diet.[53] The most recent study on fish consumption showed that consumption of more than one fatty fish meal a week was associated with a 52 percent lower risk of sudden cardiac death compared with consumption of less than one fish meal per month.[54]

Olive oil and the Omega-3 oils—canola, walnut and flaxseed—have been medically proven to lower blood pressure. In one study women with moderately high blood pressure switched to olive oil for a month and had significant drops in blood pressure.[55]

Omega-3 fatty acids also increase production of nitric oxide, which relaxes your arteries.[56] In addition, Omega-3 fatty acids seem to behave as aspirin does, acting against inflammation. They reduce the number of white blood cells that respond to inflammation, thereby reducing the risk of chronic inflammation.[57]

Omega-3 fatty acids have also been linked to lower incidence of attention-deficit disorder in children and less hostile attitudes in adults.[58]

The current consensus is that eating fish is beneficial at surprisingly modest intakes. The benefit probably depends on the fatty acid profile of the fish. There does not appear to be a greater reduction in the risk of heart disease death, especially sudden deaths, in those who ate fatty fish more than once or twice per week.[59]

People who are unable to eat fish or shellfish can take fish oil supplements. For primary prevention, 2–3 grams of fish oil per day is desirable. Higher doses should be used for prevention of a second heart attack.

EATING RIGHT FOR LONG LIFE

A heart can beat forever under ideal conditions. Nobody can live forever, but it is within your power and mine to lengthen our lives, God willing, by eating right. Just as God makes us stewards of money, talents and relationships, He makes us stewards of our bodies, and I believe He rewards people who take care of their bodies with long life and health.

It takes decades for heart disease to creep up, and the food we eat during those years can make the difference in avoiding a heart attack. Doctors, drugs and technology may bail us out, but they can provide no cure, only a plumbing job. By the time you subject yourself to the medical mill of currently fashionable treatments, you have already gambled with the outcome. Proper dietary changes can keep you healthy without interventions, surgeries or chemicals. But if your arteries are in really bad shape, don't worry; do the plumbing, and then start to clean up your act.

If more people practiced prevention in their diet and other lifestyle habits, life spans would lengthen and heart disease would not be nearly as common as it is today. According to the National Center for Health Statistics, if all forms of heart disease were eliminated, the average life span would rise by almost ten years. If all forms of cancer were eliminated, the gain would be only three years.

In fact, heart disease should not take any lives at all. I believe the vast majority of deaths due to heart disease are preventable by changing lifestyle habits.

In the next chapter I want to talk about other aspects of a heart-healthy diet. The steps we will look at are ones you can adopt today. They don't require seeing a physician, and they are far more cost-effective than any treatment.

Chapter 6

Choosing a Heart-Smart Eating Lifestyle

D o you have a friend who likes to disagree with everything you say? The kind of person who takes pleasure in refuting your beliefs—just to get your reaction?

I have a friend like that—my best friend, in fact. This friend loves to point out that many people enjoy long and healthy lives while eating junk foods and fancy French cuisine. George Bernard Shaw said, "There is no more sincere love than the love of food." My friend is living proof of that. He is bent on proving his own theory that junk food is OK and disproving my idea that diet greatly impacts health.

We do agree on some points, though barely. He agrees that exercise is important, so he plays golf. I refuse to call golf exercise, especially since my friend doesn't walk from green to green but drives a cart.

And though it may sound like boasting, I am in much better shape than he is. We both enjoy skiing, but after a couple of runs he has to take a break. He doesn't have the stamina to ski every day, but at age forty-nine, five years older than my friend, I can ski from the time they open the lifts until they close—every day! My friend and many other friends I have feel chest pains after minimal physical effort. I can run up the four flights of stairs to my office and still have tremendous energy.

I try to keep my body in good shape. My friend does not worry too much about the extra pounds he carries, and the only thing he keeps in perfect "shape" is his rounded belly. Still, he likes to point out that the only way we will know who is right about junk food, he or I, is by seeing who dies first. He actually believes that he will be present at my funeral.

I have to admit: I don't know for sure that I will live longer than my friend, but I would not exchange my lifestyle for any another. I am going to keep eating right because I know for a fact that life can be lengthened and enhanced if a person improves his or her diet.

SAYING "NO"

A big part of improving our diet is avoiding foods that harm our hearts. Today that means rejecting much of what is considered normal by society at large: popcorn slathered in butter, fast-food hamburgers, French fries and many supermarket snacks. These are unhealthy because they contain so much fat and so little nutritional value.

But foods also become unhealthy when they are processed, preserved and chemicalized to the point where they are hardly foods at all, but rather manufactured products that happen to be somewhat digestible.

In this chapter I want to discuss some common foods that are bad for the heart. They fall into several categories:

- Refined sugar
- Salt
- Refined flour
- Processed oils
- Pesticides
- Fertilized foods
- Seasonally manipulated foods
- Hormone-injected foods

Let's look at some foods to avoid and see why they are harmful to us.

REFINED SUGAR

If you had to guess which three foods are the staple of the American diet, what would you say they are? The answer is:

- Refined sugar
- Refined flour
- Processed oils

These three ingredients form the basis of most of what the average American eats. Every cracker, cereal, pastry, fruit bar and most other snacks are made up of refined sugar, refined flour

> A big part of improving our diet is avoiding foods that harm our hearts.

and processed oil. Do an experiment: Go into your pantry and look at the ingredients on the bags or boxes of food. You might be surprised how often these "three amigos" turn up.

Refined sugar is perhaps the most consumed food on the planet. Everything from fruit juice to candy bars to canned corn is sweetened with it. Think for a moment of what you have eaten today already. In all likelihood you have met your FDA-recommended sugar intake and have eaten several foods that contain white flour and processed oils.

Refined sugar is relatively new to the world scene, invented in 1751. Back then nobody ate refined sugar. Today the average American eats about 150 pounds per year, per person—about half a pound a day![1] Imagine yourself sitting in front of a bowl containing 8 ounces of pure, white sugar, and you will get an idea of how much the average American eats every day.

Refined sugar is created when raw sugar is stripped of any substances that cause it to decompose. The sweet part of the sugar remains, but anything of value is gone. In fact, nutritionists call it an "antinutrient" because our bodies waste nutrients turning it into something usable.

What does this have to do with the heart? There is a direct relationship between the explosion of heart disease in this century and the skyrocketing consumption of refined foods, including sugar. A diet that consists mainly of sugar can bring on many illnesses and is believed to increase the risk of heart attacks.[2]

It has been shown that people who eat less sugar live longer. The Seventh-Day Adventists, for example, eat a vegetarian diet and avoid refined foods. It is no coincidence that they live an average of twelve years longer than the rest of the population.

Should we rule out all sweets? No. Nature provides a wonderful sweetener called honey, a naturally occurring, unrefined sweetener that tastes every bit as good as sugar and won't harm our hearts.

I suggest replacing refined sugar with honey as often as you can. You can bake with honey, pour it into coffee or tea and spread it on bread. It has a rich, complex, sweet taste that makes refined sugar seem almost childish. You will enjoy it immensely, I assure you.

SALT

The history of salt is long, covering thousands of years and encompassing religion, economics, wars, political battles and now health and disease. Early civilization was concerned with finding and conserving salt. It was so precious that social bonds were formed over it.[3]

Because salt is abundant in our diet and because we cannot always depend on its taste to warn us of overindulgence, we need to focus on how much to consume rather than on its availability. Most of our salt intake comes from processed food, where salt is used as a preservative and often cannot be tasted.[4] Only 20 to 30 percent of total dietary sodium consumption is discretionary—or consumer-controlled—through the addition of salt to food after its preparation. The rest is derived from naturally occurring sources or commercial processes.

> There is a direct relationship between the explosion of heart disease in this century and the skyrocketing consumption of refined foods, including sugar.

Hypertension plays an important role in the development of myocardial infarction, cerebrovascular accidents, congestive heart failure and renal failure. The question of whether restricting dietary salt can prevent primary hypertension and whether a low-salt diet really helps in the treatment of hypertension is still controversial.[5]

Restriction of salt intake for the general population is not recommended at present because there is not enough evidence that this would reduce hypertension.[6] To avoid excessive intake of salt, choose foods low in salt (e.g., fresh fruits and vegetables), avoid foods high in salt (e.g., pre-prepared foods) and be aware of the salt content of food choices in restaurants.[7]

Otherwise, for hypertensive patients, particularly those who are over the age of forty-four years, obese, blacks and women, it is recommended that the intake of dietary sodium be moderately restricted to a range of 1.2–2.4 grams per day (which corresponds to 3–6 grams of salt per day).[8]

If you are hypertensive, it is important to talk with your doctor about how much salt you take in.[9]

REFINED FLOUR

We saw in the previous chapter how healthy grain and fiber are for the heart. But we don't get all the benefits from wheat because most of it is refined. When grain is refined and turned into white flour, it loses nearly all of its nutrients, and the number of calories goes up by 7 percent! White flour is almost a nonfood, stripped of nutritional value.

Even "enriched" breads are not truly healthy. They contain a few added vitamins and minerals, but not nearly enough to make up for what was lost in refining.

Worse, refined flour and white breads are treated with chemicals and bleach that get inside our arteries and cause damage. You would do well to eliminate refined flours from your diet as much as you can. Whole-grain alternatives are readily available, as we saw in the last chapter.

PROCESSED OILS

You have probably seen the words *partially hydrogenated vegetable oil* on a product in your cupboard or refrigerator. Partial hydrogenation is a process of heating vegetable oils to change the chemical constitution, producing a fat that is solid at room temperature. Margarine and shortenings are examples. Many foods, particularly snack foods, contain partially hydrogenated fats.

Foods made with partially hydrogenated fats last longer than foods made with animal fats and are less expensive. Yet these chemical substances can't be metabolized by our body. Even worse, they block our body's use of essential oils.

Processed oils have been shown to increase the risk of heart disease. A study in a major medical journal said that, "Given the proper incentives, the food industry could replace a large proportion of the partially hydrogenated fats used in foods and food preparation with unhydrogenated oils. Such a change would substantially

> The question of whether restricting dietary salt can prevent primary hypertension and whether a low-salt diet really helps in the treatment of hypertension is still controversial.

107

reduce the risk of coronary heart disease at a moderate cost."[10]

You should avoid processed oils and any foods with "partially hydrogenated oil" on their label. Substitute olive oil and butter for margarine and Crisco. Leave the chemicals for the cleaning supply cabinet, not the pantry.

PESTICIDES

The food industry hates bugs and wages war on them with pesticides. As a result, American consumers have grocery stores lined with plastic-looking fruit that lasts weeks rather than days. In truth, "buggy" fruit is not really a threat to our health. Washing and cooking it takes care of the problem.

But pesticides are a huge public health threat. Mounting evidence says that exposure to pesticides can cause cancer and other degenerative diseases. I am certain that some day tests will show a connection between heart disease and pesticides because of the damage these chemicals inflict on the lining of our arteries.

When food is treated with chemicals, those chemicals get inside our bodies and inflame the lining of our arteries, causing them to harden. It takes years, decades, even lifetimes to rid the body of these chemicals.

Instead of buying the strange-looking, too-perfect fruit and vegetables at the supermarket, seek out a store that sells pesticide-free produce. Look for the organic label. That way you can avoid putting those bug poisons in your bloodstream.

FERTILIZERS

Fertilizers also damage the foods we eat. To grow the vegetables and fruits bigger and faster, growers dump indiscriminate amounts of fertilizers into the soil, and as soon as the harvest is done, the soil is prepared for the next crop. The nutritional value of the fruits and vegetables is dramatically diminished. The most frequently used fertilizers destroy iron, vitamin C, folic acid, minerals, lysine and many other amino acids, among other nutrients.

The biblical wisdom about how to treat the soil should be learned well by today's growers:

> Six years you shall sow your field, and six years you shall prune your vineyard, and gather its fruit; but in the seventh year there shall be a sabbath of solemn rest for the land, a sabbath to the LORD. You shall neither sow your field nor prune your vineyard. What grows of its own accord of your harvest you shall not reap, nor gather the grapes of your untended vine, for it is a year of rest for the land.
>
> —LEVITICUS 25:3–5

If land were allowed to rest, it would retain its ability to give nutrition. Instead, growers use fields year round, in and out of the natural season, and would never consider giving their fields an entire year off.

Again, eating organically grown, fertilizer-free produce will help you to get the heart-healthy nutrients you need and avoid the questionable chemicals that come with the fertilizer.

SEASONALLY MANIPULATED FOODS

To increase shelf life, farmers harvest fruits and vegetables long before they are mature, even though produce absorbs most of its vitamins and minerals when it is almost ripe.

Today's farmers ignore the biblical wisdom of seasons. It

was Solomon who said, "To everything there is a season, a time for every purpose under heaven…A time to plant, and a time to pluck what is planted" (Eccles. 3:1–2).

> I am certain that some day tests will show a connection between heart disease and pesticides because of the damage these chemicals inflict on the lining of our arteries.

There is a time to plant and a time to pluck the fruit. This means that there is also a time not to pluck the fruit. But modern agriculture demands that the season be always now.

Green bananas will never fill up with vitamins and minerals sitting on your kitchen counter! Potatoes lose most of their vitamin C in a week, and spinach greens, asparagus, broccoli and peas lose half of their vitamins before they get to market.

Packaging and transportation compromises nutritional value even more. If picked and left outside more than two or three hours, nutritional value is further reduced.

Frozen vegetables lose one-fourth of vitamins A, B_1, B_2, C and niacin. Broccoli, cauliflower, peas and spinach lose up to half of their vitamins. Canned foods lose more than half of all nutrients—but provide a substantial amount of lead!

Eating fresh, organically grown produce is the best way to get nutrients. Seek out a farmer's market and inquire about their growing methods. Ask if they let their fields rest and if they use pesticides or fertilizers. With the growing popularity of organic foods, such heart-healthy produce shouldn't be hard to find.

HORMONE-INJECTED FOODS

Another major source of questionable chemicals is animal products. Fifty years ago, a dairy cow produced two thousand pounds of milk per year. Today the average cow gives fifty thousand pounds of milk per year. How is such a radical increase possible? Only with the assistance of hormones.

You may think that milk is just milk, but the FDA allows milk producers to give their cows up to eighty-two different drugs. These drugs never make it onto the nutrition facts label. The milk you drink is swimming in hormones. Two of the most-used—bovine growth hormone and estrogen—are believed to have a synergistic effect that provokes heart disease.

Cows bred for slaughter are also injected with growth hormones so they grow bigger faster. Meat has been known to contain up to fourteen times the amount of pesticides and other chemicals as in plant foods.[11]

At health food supermarkets you can choose from a variety of milks that are produced without hormones. I encourage you to buy and enjoy the pure stuff to enhance your heart health.

A WORD ABOUT "LITE" AND "LOW-FAT" FOODS

One of the biggest jokes the food industry plays is that "lite" and "low-fat" foods are good for you. Nothing could be further from the truth! These labels typically mean the product has less fat than the regular version. I have seen "lite" candy bars and even "lite" Twinkies!

But harmful chemicals, preservatives and food colorings remain in the foods, along with large amounts of refined sugar, refined flour and processed oils. Nothing healthy has been added.

Lately the push is on to produce fake fats—essentially plastics—that decrease the calories people absorb from fat. Nabisco launched a product with the texture of fat, "salatrim," for its cookies. The NutraSweet company put imitation ice creams and sherbets on the market, but because their texture was not pleasing to the palate, they stopped producing them. A synthetic fat is used in some frozen desserts and in some cheeses and mayonnaise.

> Eating fresh, organically grown produce is the best way to get nutrients.

A few years ago the FDA allowed Procter & Gamble to try out a fake fat called Olestra. It passes through the digestive tract without being digested or absorbed, much as gum does when swallowed. The company put it in several products, including potato chips. Olestra caused diahrrea in some people and stomach cramps in others.

But a greater concern with fake fats is that some day they will be found to have harmful long-term effects. Common sense tells us that there are no foods without consequences. Nutritious foods have healthy consequences. Non-nutritious foods have harmful consequences. Either they leave a residue of strange chemicals in our bodies, or they block our intestines from absorbing good things. I am reminded that for many years the medical industry said that cigarettes were healthy. What will they say about these fake fats, processed foods and hormone-rich meat in twenty years?

The "lite" and "low-fat" labels should be looked on with skepticism. After all, if these foods were helping us be healthier, why are people still getting fatter and fatter?

NON-MANIPULATED FOODS

Chemicals introduced by the tremendous manipulation of our foodstuffs cause heart disease. The best diets are those in which the food is not laden with chemical preservatives, drugs and hormones; the food is not packaged, canned, frozen, precooked, processed or genetically altered or has not sat on a supermarket shelf for months.

Go for fresh, fragrant, bursting-with-flavor foods that were recently harvested, slaughtered or milked. You will notice a dramatic difference in their flavor, and your heart will be free of the strange or questionable chemicals that could harden your arteries.

One of the basic principles of biblical prevention wisdom is this: Eat foods close to the way they were put on earth.

CHOOSING THE PRIMITIVE DIET

Can you imagine living in a day with no airplanes, automobiles, televisions, radios or computers?

Can you imagine living, as they did a hundred years ago, under the threat of various diseases, viruses and plagues that would sweep through a community and kill thousands?

Today we have so many mind-boggling technologies and medicines to keep sickness at bay and to make life easier. I

113

am thankful for all of the modern marvels—but when it comes to food, I am as old-fashioned as they come.

I believe that the best diet on the planet is the one people ate until the twentieth century—a primitive diet based on what the land produced, what grew in the garden, what the cow gave in the way of milk and what the herd gave in the way of fresh meat.

The primitive diet means eating things close to how they naturally occur. People who eat primitive diets generally:

- Do not have heart disease
- Do not have cavities or gum disease
- Do not gain weight as they age
- Have low blood pressure
- Are physically fit

There was a dentist in the early part of this century who decided to travel the world to fulfill his wanderlust. His name was Weston Price. Instead of sticking to the well-trod vacation paths in Europe and America, he ventured into then-uncivilized places: the forests and jungles in Asia.

Price couldn't help his curiosity when he met people from relatively primitive tribes. He studied the people and found that they did not have the problems with degenerative diseases like heart disease and cancer that Westernized people did.[12]

Price, being a dentist, counted cavities and found that less than 1 percent of the people's teeth were decayed. He found some groups in which tooth decay was actually nonexistent. None of these people brushed their teeth or visited dentists.[13]

Price discovered what other researchers have discovered:

People who eat primitive diets not only avoid Western diseases like cancer and even gum disease, but they also virtually never have heart disease.

BACK TO BETTER WAYS

When I began studying the primitive diet, I realized that here is a way to make lifestyle changes that have been proven over many centuries in many parts of the world to prevent heart disease. It is not a silver bullet, but it is as close as we can come.

For example, among the Kitava, a primitive people in Papua New Guinea, heart attacks, strokes and chest pain are virtually nonexistent. All the adults have low blood pressure and are lean. But when a Kitava person adopts the Western diet, his health changes. One middle-aged Kitava man who moved to the city and became a businessman was found to have higher blood pressure and more body fat than the ones at home.[14]

> One of the basic principles of biblical prevention wisdom is this: Eat foods close to the way they were put on earth.

A group of aboriginal Australians virtually recovered from diabetes in five weeks by returning to their traditional diet. And a group of obese Hawaiians lost an average of five pounds each in three weeks eating their traditional foods in whatever quantity they wanted, and without exercising![15]

In China, a study showed that Chinese people who shift to a Western diet increase their risk of heart disease and stroke, whereas villagers in rural Chinese villages have the lowest rates of heart disease in the world. The typical village diet consists of very little meat, steamed rice, vegetables and steamed fish or tofu. The incidence of heart disease is incredibly low.

By contrast, the Chinese who live in the modern cities eat much more meat, dairy products and ice cream and have higher rates of heart disease.[16]

These are just a few examples, but they make it clear: Eating the types of foods we have looked at in the previous chapters can actually keep heart disease at bay.

THE MEDITERRANEAN DIET

Recall the last time you visited an Italian restaurant. As you waited for your meal you probably munched on buttered bread while watching the waiter go by with trays of pasta drenched with cream sauces, meat sauces and cheese.

That is a far cry from what real Mediterranean food is. Real Italians eat pasta with very little meat. They use meat and cheese sparingly, the way Americans use relish.

In its essence, the real Mediterranean diet is the closest thing the Western world has to a primitive diet—and it has wide-ranging health benefits.

But in Italian restaurants all over the U.S. dishes are loaded down with fatty sauces and meats. Standard restaurant dishes like fettuccine Alfredo are often laden with as much saturated fat as three pints of butter almond ice cream! And a serving of fried calamari may have as much cholesterol as a four-egg omelet![17]

The term *Mediterranean diet* refers to dietary patterns found in olive-growing areas of the Mediterranean region, where culture integrates the past and the present.

The traditional Mediterranean diet has eight components:

- High monounsaturated/saturated fat ratio, principally from olive oil
- Moderate alcohol consumption, principally from red wine and almost always during meals
- High consumption of legumes
- High consumption of whole grains and cereals, including bread
- High consumption of fruits
- High consumption of vegetables
- Low consumption of meat and meat products
- Moderate consumption of milk and dairy products[18]

Healthcare for many of Mediterranean populations was inferior to that available to people in northern Europe and U.S. However, death rates in the Mediterranean region were generally lower and adult life expectancy generally higher compared with the more economically developed countries of Europe and North America, particularly among men.[19] A dramatic lower incidence of myocardial infarction and death was reported in patients consuming the Mediterranean-type diet.[20]

The real Mediterranean diet is very healthy and is associated with low risk of heart disease. The usual ingredients are:

- Fresh fish
- Steamed vegetables
- Olive oil
- Wine
- Fresh fruit

If you stick with these basic foods, you will be eating the time-honored primitive diet, and your heart will fall in love with you all over again.

CHANGE FROM THE HEART

> The real Mediterranean diet is the closest thing the Western world has to a primitive diet—and it has wide-ranging health benefits.

Changing diets as much as I am recommending—buying organic foods, avoiding processed foods, eating fresh things and avoiding preservatives—may seem difficult, but it is the only sensible way to gain greater heart health.

Some day, perhaps not long from now, eating chemically processed, nutritionally vacuous food will be seen as a health hazard, and most of what stocks the shelves of grocery stores will be a thing of the past. Until then, be aggressive with your health and your diet. Set the pace for healthy living, and your heart will reward you with a long and active life.

Chapter 7

Boost Heart Power With Supplements, Aspirin and Hormones

S usan is fifty-one years old, a new grandmother and part-time consultant at a publicity firm. With her children in college and a burgeoning second career, she is content. But the nagging memory of her father's death by heart attack still haunts her, and she has started looking into ways of reducing her own risk.

She has heard and read a lot about vitamin, mineral and herb supplements that can help prevent heart disease, so she went to the drugstore to buy some, but she wasn't sure which one was heart-healthiest. She scanned the aisles for a while, then settled for a bottle of multivitamins, but still unsure what benefit she would reap from it and whether she should go further and buy some of the herbal remedies she saw.

But if so, which ones? There were so many...

She has also read a magazine article about aspirin and its wonderful effect on circulation and the heart, but the article seemed to indicate that aspirin mainly helped men. *Should I take aspirin?* she wonders, *How often? How much?*

Finally, she has heard about aggressive preventive measures especially for women. Susan has gone through menopause, and recently her doctor recommended taking estrogen to avoid heart disease. There are side effects, she knows. She might gain weight, and her husband, who has done a lot of research on the Internet, keeps bringing her articles that point to a connection between estrogen and breast cancer. Susan's doctor mentioned this during their consultation, but he indicated that the benefits of taking estrogen outweighed the possible side effects.

Was he right? Susan isn't sure, but it is a small price to pay, she thinks, to keep a heart attack from spoiling her life. If that means taking vitamins, minerals, herb supplements, aspirin and hormones, then that's what she wants to do.

WHAT TO TAKE?

Drugstores and supermarkets are full of supplement choices these days—and not just vitamins and minerals, but a host of homeopathic supplements, too. The herbal revolution is well underway.

But which supplements should we take specifically to ward off heart disease? And what about aspirin and hormone replacement therapy? Are they of any benefit? In this chapter I will give the answers. I will also discuss the latest critically important research on hormone replacement therapy.

VITAMINS

Even if you eat healthy foods, you should supplement your diet with vitamins. The American Heart Association says that taking multivitamins could prevent fifty thousand-heart disease deaths per year.[1]

"Users of multivitamins have been reported to have reduced the prevalence of coronary artery disease compared with nonusers," said doctors for the American Heart Association.[2]

Let's go through some of the best supplements for our hearts and arteries.

B vitamins

The term *niacin* is commonly used to refer to the two forms of vitamin B_3, nicotinic acid and nicotinamide. Vitamin B_3 at high doses (1.2 to 2.0 grams per day) protects against cardiovascular disease by reducing cholesterol levels as much as 22 percent, lowering triglycerides as much as 53 percent, increasing HDL-cholesterol ("good" cholesterol) by 33 percent and reducing the recurrence rate for heart attacks by almost 30 percent. Research has shown that vitamin B_3 may be capable of actually reversing some atherosclerosis.[3]

> Even if you eat healthy foods, you should supplement your diet with vitamins.

Homocysteine is an amino acid that scrapes the inner layer of blood vessels, leading to hardening. But homocysteine is an enemy that can be fought with supplements.

Recent studies showed that intake of folic acid and vitamin B_6 above the current Recommended Dietary Allowance (RDA) may be important in the primary prevention of coronary heart disease.[4]

A research study found that men with extremely high homocysteine levels were three times more likely to have a heart attack, even when adjustments for other factors such as blood lipids were considered.[5]

The results from a very recent scientific publication in which a total of 80,082 women from the Nurses' Health Study were followed up over fourteen years showed that the risk of CHD was reduced by 31 percent in the group of women with the highest average intake of vitamin B_6 and folate, compared with the group of women with the lowest average intake of vitamin B_6 and folate.[6]

> The amount of vitamin C needed to keep a healthy heart is equal to the vitamin C found in one orange or one apple.

The current RDA for folate of 180 micrograms per day and for vitamin B_6 of 1.6 to 2.0 milligrams per day may not be sufficient to minimize the risk of coronary disease. The lowest risk observed in the studies was with intakes of folic acid above 400 micrograms per day and vitamin B_6 above 3 milligrams per day. It is estimated that 88 to 90 percent of the U.S. population has dietary intakes for folate below 400 micrograms per day. (The national average is 225 micrograms per day.) The maximum benefit would be achieved at folate intake of at least 400 micrograms per day.

The B vitamins work together as a team, which is the reason why it is generally recommended that a B-complex supplement be taken rather than the individual B vitamins.

VITAMIN C

Vitamin C is one of the most powerful heart-protecting

substances. The protective action of vitamin C has been attributed to its antioxidant effects in the prevention of oxidation of low-density lipoproteins (LDL) cholesterol ("bad" cholesterol), an early step in heart disease. Also, it decreases the "stickiness" of blood, providing additional beneficial actions, specifically in patients with coronary artery disease.[7] People who take higher doses of vitamin C are far less likely to die of heart disease and heart attacks than those who take lower doses.

"Individuals with the highest levels of vitamin C in their blood had only about half the risk of death from heart attack than those with the lowest levels," said doctors from the University of Cambridge in a recent study.[8]

The amount of vitamin C needed to keep a healthy heart is equal to the vitamin C found in one orange or one apple, so add one to your daily food schedule, perhaps in the morning or as an afternoon snack.[9] I also recommend taking a daily supplement of 2–3 grams of vitamin C, as other research points to the benefits of having larger amounts of vitamin C in the blood.

Vitamin E

Vitamin E taken in high doses has been shown to reduce the risk of heart disease by as much as 43 percent. People who take vitamin E supplements *and* cholesterol-lowering drugs show less progression of heart disease than people who take only the drugs.[10]

In one study of nearly forty thousand men, vitamin E taken daily at a dose higher than 100 International Units for two years was shown to reduce the risk of heart disease by 33 to 43 percent. Apparently, vitamin E slows down the hardening of our arteries by blocking the damaging effects of cholesterol.[11]

Keeping our body well-stocked with nutritious elements like vitamin E can slow or stop our arteries from hardening. I recommend taking a daily supplement of 400 to 800 International Units of vitamin E.

MINERALS

In addition to supplementing your diet with vitamins on a daily basis, you should also supplement with minerals and extracts that have shown healthy benefits.

CALCIUM

Low calcium intake has been linked to high blood pressure, though doctors do not know exactly why.[12] A diet moderate to high in calcium content helps reduce and prevent high blood pressure.[13] One study showed that people who eat a lot of low-fat dairy products, fruit and vegetables, thus moderate to high content (approximately 1,200 mg/day), significantly reduce their blood pressure and prevent hypertention.[14]

Calcium, of course, is found in great quantities in dairy products. I recommend drinking a moderate amount of milk or eating cheese and yogurt, making sure you stick with the low-fat versions. But do not forget that in order to absorb calcium, you must expose yourself to the sun. Most of us do not get out enough, so start enjoying walks in the park, not only on your treadmill.

CHROMIUM

Only about 0.5 percent of an oral dose of inorganic trivalent chromium is absorbed. This has led to the development of organically bonded chromium compounds, which are more cell permeable.[15] The most intriguing of these is chromium picolinate, one of the best-absorbed sources of nutritional chromium, which is formed by a molecule of trivalent chromium bonded with three molecules of organic picolinic acid.[16]

Scientific studies have shown that chromium picolinate can lower elevated low-density lipoproteins (LDL) cholesterol ("bad" cholesterol), suggesting that chromium picolinate may be useful for cardiovascular protection.[17]

I recommend 200 to 400 micrograms of chromium picolinate daily.

MAGNESIUM

Magnesium may sound like a kind of revolver or space shuttle, but it is a common and yet valuable mineral that is necessary for everything the human body does. Now a number of studies hint that magnesium has a beneficial effect on heart disease, particularly for people who have already had a heart attack.[18]

A number of research studies suggest that magnesium has a beneficial effect in ischemic heart disease and cardiac arrhythmias.[19]

This analysis concluded that available studies are strongly suggestive of magnesium's beneficial effect on mortality following acute myocardial infarction.

At present, magnesium is well accepted as a therapy for certain arrhythmias.[20] When you buy a supplement, make sure it contains magnesium.

POTASSIUM

Potassium, found in high quantities in bananas, helps our muscles to contract and our heart to beat. Potassium deficiency causes fatigue, weakness and muscle pains.

A recent study showed that eating too little potassium may

play an important role in high blood pressure. Taking potassium supplements usually can reduce your blood pressure.[21]

COENZYME Q_{10} AND AMINO ACIDS

COENZYME Q_{10}

Coenzyme Q_{10} (CoQ_{10}) is essential for the production of energy. The role of dietary CoQ_{10} intake in cardiovascular disease has been increasingly investigated. Although humans can synthesize CoQ_{10}, its levels decline as a factor of aging.[22] Smokers may be very deficient in this substance, and patients with heart disease as well.[23]

CoQ_{10} supplementation improves exercise capacity, quality of life and clinical outcome in patients with chronic congestive heart failure and in patients with acute myocardial infarction.[24] It also significantly reduces the incidence of serious complications and prolongs markedly life expectancy.[25]

For primary prevention, if you are over forty, I suggest that you take 50 milligrams daily of a commercially available form of coenzyme Q_{10} with your heaviest meal, or take 30 milligrams a day of a new fully-solubilized form of coenzyme Q_{10} (Q-Gel).

For secondary prevention, I recommend that you take 60 to 120 milligrams daily of Q-Gel (divided into two or three doses) or 200 milligrams per day of a commercial coenzyme Q_{10}.[26]

L-CARNITINE

L-carnitine plays a key role in transporting fatty acids—a major source of energy in the heart. It also protects the heart muscle against oxygen deprivation and heart attacks. Lack of this amino acid keeps the heart from beating properly.[27]

Taking L-carnitine as a supplement can help you to avoid

chest pains, irregular heartbeat, congestive heart failure, high cholesterol, heart attacks and peripheral vascular disease. It also improves stamina and endurance and increases maximal work output during exercise.[28] L-carnitine also protects the myocardium against diphtheria toxin,[29] ischemia[30] and myocardial infarction.[31]

Supplementation with L-carnitine has beneficial effects in a number of cardiovascular disorders including acute ischemia,[32] angina pectoris,[33] arrhythmias,[34] congestive heart failure,[35] hyperlipidemia[36] and after myocardial infarction,[37] as well as peripheral vascular disease.[38]

For primary prevention I recommend 0.5 to 1.0 grams of L-carnitine per day. For people who have already had a heart attack or have been diagnosed with heart failure, I recommend taking 1.0 to 2.0 grams of L-carnitine (divided into two or three doses).[39]

TAURINE

Taurine is a special amino acid found in large quantities in muscles, the brain, the heart and the blood. Taurine helps the heart muscle to contract, lowers blood pressure and is useful in treating congestive heart failure. Taurine is found in fish and shellfish.[40]

A large volume of literature is now available indicating that taurine has a unique toning action[41] and is useful in the treatment of congestive heart failure.[42] Taurine has antioxidant effects[43] and has a role regulating myocardial contraction.[44] It also lowers blood pressure[45] and strengthens heart muscle function.[46]

Taurine supplementation reduces bad cholesterol and increases HDL cholesterol ("good" cholesterol) in rats fed a high-cholesterol diet compared with rats without taurine.[47] Researchers observed a significant decrease in taurine as a result of a high-cholesterol diet.[48]

For patients with congestive heart failure or after a heart infarction, I recommend 2.0 to 3.0 grams of taurine daily (divided into two or three doses).[49]

> Taking L-carnitine as a supplement can help you to avoid chest pains, irregular heartbeat, congestive heart failure, high cholesterol, heart attacks and peripheral vascular disease.

HERBS

HAWTHORN

Fruit, flower and leaf extracts of hawthorn are known for their beneficial effects in increasing contractility of the heart muscle, improving cardiac efficiency, decreasing cholesterol blood levels and reducing blood pressure. Hawthorn has also been shown to protect the heart from damage if it is ever deprived of oxygen.[50] More doctors are using the extracts of hawthorn to treat milder forms of heart failure and to prevent a second heart attack.[51]

I recommend 300 milligrams of hawthorn extract daily. For people who already have heart trouble, I recommend 600 to 900 milligrams per day divided into two to three doses.

GRAPE SEED EXTRACT

Grape seed extract goes a long way to reduce the severity

of heart attacks and to prevent cardiovascular disease by reducing blood clots, capillary permeability and fragility and also by its antioxidant effects. I recommend taking 100 to 150 milligrams of grape seed extract per day.[52]

GINKGO BILOBA

Ginkgo biloba leaves and fruits contain substances that reduce the amount of free radicals in the blood that can harm our arteries. Ginkgo biloba also increases blood flow, especially in deeper-seated medium and small arteries in the heart muscle, and it keeps blood from becoming too sticky.[53]

I recommend taking a daily dose of 120 milligrams of a ginkgo biloba extract.

GARLIC

Garlic protects our heart in several ways. It lowers blood pressure, reduces cholesterol levels, reduces ventricular arrhythmias and prevents blood clotting. I recommend taking a daily dose equivalent to 4 grams of fresh garlic—the size of one large clove. Follow manufacturer's interactions for commercial garlic and garlic-derived products. A good range is about 900 to 1200 milligrams per day of aged garlic extract.[54]

Many of these supplements sound exotic, but one of the most popular heart attack prevention drugs on the market is probably sitting in your cupboard right now.

ASPIRIN

Aspirin has long been used to treat headaches, pains, fevers and inflammations. Now it has been proven that taking one tablet of aspirin every day decreases the number of heart attacks by as much as 40 percent.[55]

> Aspirin…has a profound effect on a component of the blood called platelets—blood cells that stick together and cause clots to form…Aspirin has been shown to be beneficial after a heart attack and for reducing the risk of a heart attack in people who suffer from unstable angina and possibly also in people who suffer from stable angina.[56]

Aspirin has also been shown to reduce the risk of stroke, which is related to heart disease. Most news reports focus on the benefit of aspirin to men, but it also helps women avoid heart problems.

> In women under age 50 with a strong family history of heart attacks at an early age, obesity, a smoking habit, or some other risk factor such as diabetes, it probably is a good idea to take one baby aspirin or one-half of a regular aspirin each day…The aspirin usually does no harm and may help prevent a heart attack.[57]

Aspirin is recommended to be taken by someone who has suffered a heart attack because it works against the artery-blocking clot. "In addition to thrombolytic agents, aspirin and heparin may also be administered. These drugs can prevent a clot in the artery from growing larger or from reforming after it has been dissolved by the thrombolytic agent."[58]

However, "William Lee Cowden, M.D., a cardiologist from Dallas, Texas suggests that this approach may be misguided, since aspirin has been shown to cause gastrointestinal bleeding and even perforated ulcers…"[59] To avoid aspirin's side effects I recommend taking Omega 3 fatty acids.

There is one more type of "supplement" to talk about, and it deals exclusively with women and a procedure called Hormone Replacement Therapy, or HRT.

HORMONE REPLACEMENT THERAPY

For many years, doctors have been prescribing HRT for post-menopausal women like Susan. Heart disease in women increases significantly in the years after menopause, and doctors assumed this was due to the drop in hormone levels. To counter the drop, doctors prescribed estrogen or estrogen-progesterone replacements to try to reduce the incidence of heart disease.

Not only did HRT replace the missing hormones, but it also increased "good" cholesterol and decreased "bad" cholesterol. For years the benefits of HRT were virtually unassailable in the medical community.

But three major trials designed to prove the heart-healthy benefits of HRT have, so far, failed to do so. In one study, the women taking HRT had an increase of heart attacks, strokes and blood clots.

> Aspirin has long been used to treat headaches, pains, fevers and inflammations. Now it has been proven that taking one tablet of aspirin every day decreases the number of heart attacks.

If you are a woman and your doctor has prescribed HRT for the prevention of heart disease, I strongly disagree with

131

the recommendation. HRT is now discredited as a treatment for heart disease, and it might actually be a cause. Most of the same doctors who once prescribed it out of hand now find no reason to do so.

I cannot see any reason to prescribe HRT for menopausal women when changes in lifestyle do much more to prevent heart disease. The fact that it increases the incidence of breast cancer should make HRT totally unacceptable.

Unfortunately, today heart disease is a woman's disease as much as a man's. But by careful attention to eating and exercise habits, women can beat the rap and avoid living in its shadow—without HRT.

> Taking the right kinds of supplements—vitamins, minerals, natural extracts and aspirin—will supply your heart with the ammunition needed to fight heart disease.

Taking the right kinds of supplements—vitamins, minerals, natural extracts and aspirin—will supply your heart with the ammunition needed to fight heart disease. It's an investment worth making the next time you go to the drugstore.

Chapter 8

Weighing In
for Heart Health

The man walked into the seafood restaurant with every intention of taking them up on their "all-you-can-eat" offer, embarking on an eating binge that left the other patrons and the restaurant staff stunned.

He began to load two plates at a time with hot, steaming crab legs and Chinese cuisine. When he was finished, he went back to the food bar and loaded up two more plates. The cook in the back began to wonder why there was so much demand for crab legs—he couldn't seem to make them fast enough.

Soon, the employees and customers started noticing the man's appetite. Other patrons were getting angry because there was no food left for them.

The server brought his bill as a not-so-subtle hint, but he kept right on eating. They brought a second bill, adding ten dollars to the total for "snow crab." He kept on eating.

Finally, he took the first bill to the register where the waiter insisted he pay the additional money because he had eaten so much. He refused, and an argument broke out that only stopped when the local sheriff stepped in. The sheriff sided with the man: All-you-can-eat meant all-you-can-eat, no matter how much it cost the restaurant.[1]

That may not be a common scene, but it actually happened, and in small ways it happens every day. People go to McDonald's or a sit-down restaurant and order food until they literally can't eat anymore. The result is a population of overweight, out of shape, heart-diseased people who measure their enjoyment by how many plates they can empty.

Heart disease is caused not just by what we eat, but also how much. For all the fretting and fad-dieting Americans do, we are one of the fattest countries on the planet.

If you go to a mall in China, Egypt or Singapore, you have to look long and hard to find overweight people. But malls in America are crowded with overweight people—and not just the pudgy, but the morbidly fat.

A startling graphic in a magazine not long ago showed that in 1991 four U.S. states had populations that were considered dangerously obese, meaning 15 percent of the population was fat. Ten years later, forty-four states have dangerously obese populations! Virtually the entire country is considered over the line of healthy weight.[2]

Surveys paint a troubling portrait. More than half of the U.S. population is overweight, and that number is rising. More than one quarter of Americans are not just fat, but excessively fat.[3]

Each year, the number of obese people increases by 6 percent—about fifteen million people. The number of fat people in their thirties has grown at 10 percent per year.

"As obesity rates continue to grow at epidemic proportions in this country, the net effect will be dramatic increases in related chronic health conditions such as diabetes and cardio-vascular disease in the future," said a doctor with the Centers for Disease Control and Prevention.[4]

But most Americans deny they have a weight problem.[5] They prefer to think they are "pleasantly plump," or just have a "spare tire," or are still working off fat from a pregnancy. And when you look around and see so many other fat people, obesity begins to seem normal.

But obesity is not normal to the human body. It is a legitimate, epidemic health threat. The Surgeon General warned a decade ago that "for most of us the problem has become one of overeating—too many calories for our activity levels and an imbalance in the nutrients consumed along with them."[6]

That certainly describes many Americans. We eat far more calories than we expend, and those calories pile up in the form of unsightly fat. Not only that, but our forms of entertainment— watching television, attending a sporting event, playing video games—don't require much energy.

> Heart disease is caused not just by what we eat, but also how much.

Our occupations also put a damper on our activity levels. A century ago, farmers, machine-builders, railroad workers, blacksmiths and textile workers all relied on the energy produced by their muscles. Today every task from the biggest to the smallest is accomplished by pushing a button and letting electricity- or steam-powered machines do the heavy lifting.

Think about it: When was the last time you huffed and puffed because of physical exertion at your job?

135

Those factors have made obesity the most common and costly nutritional problem in the U.S., and it costs us not just in food bills or public shame but in medical bills. Healthcare costs directly caused by obesity amount to $68 billion per year; an additional $30 billion per year is spent on weight-reduction programs and special foods. Nevertheless, treatments intended to slim people down are largely ineffective, and 90 to 95 percent of persons who lose weight regain it. If you have been in the diet mill, you know what that feels like.

This is a good time to ask yourself the following questions: Are you overweight? By how much? Do you have an honest assessment of yourself? Have you tried every fad under the sun? Every pill advertised in the back of health magazines? Maybe it's time for you to see it not just as a "look great, feel great" issue, but a matter of saving your own life.

OBESITY AND THE HEART

Obesity is one of the most common and reversible causes of heart disease. Being overweight is linked to more than three hundred thousand premature deaths each year in the United States, second only to tobacco-related deaths.[7]

Studies have found that excess body weight increases the risk of death from heart disease and virtually every other ailment.[8] In studies of men and women, overweight people had a 50 to 72 percent greater chance of a heart attack than people who were not overweight.[9]

Like any imbalance in the body, excess weight acts like the first domino in a series of problems. It raises your blood pressure, raises cholesterol levels and can bring on diabetes.[10]

What qualifies as overweight? The rule of thumb is that a

waist circumference over 40 inches in men and over 35 inches in women increases the risk for heart disease and other diseases.[11]

But there are more exact ways of assessing your weight, the most widely being the Body Mass Index (BMI). This compares height with weight and gives you a rough idea if you are overweight and at risk. I'll show you how to figure your BMI in a moment. First, the figures: People with a BMI from 18.5 to around 25 are considered healthy. People with a BMI between 25 and 30 are considered overweight and at moderate risk for heart problems. People with a BMI over 30 are considered at high risk.

Here's what you do. Weigh yourself on a scale, making sure to wear light clothing and no shoes. Then measure your height to the nearest quarter inch.

> Healthcare costs directly caused by obesity amount to $68 billion per year; an additional $30 billion per year is spent on weight-reduction programs and special foods.

Now comes the math: Multiply your weight by 705 (don't ask why—it's just part of the formula). If you weigh 155 pounds you would do this:

155 x 705 = 109,275

That's not your BMI! Next, divide that number by your height in inches. If you are five feet five inches, your height in inches is 65 and your equation would look like this:

$$109,275 \div 65 = 1681$$

Then take 1681 and divide it by your height in inches one more time:

$$1681 \div 65 = 25.86$$

That is your BMI. Here is the formula: Multiply your weight in pounds by 705. Divide that number by your height in inches. Then divide by your height in inches again to get your BMI.

Remember, the desired range is a BMI of 25 or less. A person with a BMI between 25 and 30 is considered overweight and has a moderate risk of heart disease. Any BMI above 30 is considered dangerous.

> We owe it to ourselves and to the people who love us to manage our weight responsibly.

As you can see, the sample person we used—five feet five inches and 155 pounds—has a BMI in the overweight, moderate risk category. The ideal weight for such a person would be 149 pounds or less. The danger zone would be 180 pounds or more.[11]

But it's not just your weight relative to your height that counts. It's how that weight is distributed. If you are a woman with extra weight in your hips or thighs, that is not nearly as heart-risky as having extra weight on your abdomen.[12]

Put plainly, people with pear-shaped bodies, with the bulk of the weight at or below the waistline, are at less risk than people with apple-shaped bodies, where the weight is carried between the neck and waist.[13] If you tend to have an apple shape, you should take the threat of heart disease very seriously and work to get your BMI into an acceptable range.

Of course, each of us is built differently, but wherever extra fat is carried—around your middle, under your arms, in the backs of your thighs—it acts like an anchor on your heart, causing it to work harder to push blood through the body. It is high time we stop blaming our excess weight on being "big-boned" or "meaty." Shifting the blame may cost us years of life, and we owe it to ourselves and to the people who love us to manage our weight responsibly.

KIDS AND HEART DISEASE

Obesity and heart disease begin in childhood. By age twelve, as many as 70 percent of children have fatty deposits in their arteries, which is a step away from developing hard arteries.[14]

The Bogalusa Heart Study, the longest and most detailed study of children in the world, found that the major signs of heart disease can be detected in children as young as five years old. Another study found damage in the hearts of subjects as young as three years old.[15] That is remarkable—and remarkably frightening. Autopsy studies on children have shown lesions in the aorta, coronary vessels and kidney, indicating hard arteries and high blood pressure.[16]

Children are literally suffering from heart disease before they enter the first grade!

Does this mean that twelve-year-olds are going to start dying of heart attacks? Probably not. Heart disease takes years to develop. But by the time a young person hits his or her teenage years, chances are good that he or she has real arterial damage.

One of the primary contributors to artery damage in children is obesity. As many as one in four children between the ages of six and seventeen is overweight, which comes as no surprise to anyone who works with children or simply sees the number of overweight kids in public places.[17]

Obese children grow up to be at-risk adults. People who were fat as children have a much greater chance of having heart attacks than adults who were not obese as children. Heart trouble can even be predicted by the body shape—apple or pear—of children as young as nine years old.[18]

Obviously, eating well and keeping our weight down should start when we are children. In a way, parents are to blame for burdening their children with unhealthy diets and excess fat. Kids "learn" obesity through the habits passed on to them. Most kids today load up on unhealthy foods, or they overeat, or both. Whole families spend Sunday's noon hour at a fast-food place or an "all-you-can-eat" restaurant gorging themselves on one tempting dish after another, like the scene I described in the beginning of this chapter?

It is not uncommon for parents to push their children to keep eating, even when the child is inclined to stop. Sometimes parents want to get their money's worth for a meal, or they stuff the kids full so they don't say "I'm hungry" for the rest of the day. Sometimes they simply give the child adult portions.

All those practices are wrong. Overweight children are at-risk children. Putting pounds on as a kid is like putting the welcome mat out for heart disease.

On the other hand, children who jog or play sports are more likely to be fit and less likely to be fat.[19] And healthy habits in childhood clearly can stop the hardening of arteries.

"Weight control, and encouragement of physical exercise and a prudent diet, if undertaken early in life, may retard the [hardening of the arteries]," wrote one doctor in a major study of heart disease in children.[20]

Some parents don't change their kids' habits because they fear it will inflict psychological trauma. What would little Susie do, after all, without her McNuggets? But studies show that changes in a child's diet will not harm him or her in any way—emotionally, spiritually or socially. Teaching a child to treat his or her body correctly leads to greater health, well-being, energy and stamina.[21]

"Heart-healthy diets appeared to be brain-friendly as well," the report said. "After three years on the diet, the children [placed on a healthier diet] had lowered their cholesterol levels but no adverse effects in terms of academic function were evident, nor were there differences in psychological symptoms or family functioning."

> Children are literally suffering from heart disease before they enter the first grade!

Obesity in kids is not "cute." I have heard too many parents say, "My child isn't fat; he just has a healthy appetite." A truly healthy appetite keeps weight at a proper level. The healthiest appetites tell you when to stop eating. There is nothing healthy about being fat.

Our nation is raising a generation of fat kids who will have a rude awakening as they move through adulthood. Their risk for heart disease will be greater even than the risk in the present generation of adults. Heart disease might be a greater threat to our children than it is to us—if we continue to hand down wrong habits.

Children should learn moderation, not gluttony, from their parents. Everyone else around them may teach them to eat until drowsy, to indulge, to take as much as they can—but wouldn't it be nice if they saw you controlling your appetite? Exercising to keep weight off? Saying "no" to seconds and thirds?

> Teaching a child to treat his or her body correctly leads to greater health, well-being, energy and stamina.

It's one sure way you can add years to your child's life.

If you or your loved ones are victims of obesity, start seeing it as a health issue. Instead of getting on the diet merry-go-round, make basic changes and stick with them.

- ॐ Eat the kinds of foods we talked about in the food chapter.
- ॐ Don't overeat. You can get fat by eating too much of the right foods.
- ॐ Limit the times and places you allow yourself to eat.
- ॐ Don't snack yourself to a higher waist size.
- ॐ Incorporate other life changes like exercising (which we will talk about in the next chapter).

Don't let fat determine your fate! Guard your heart from the dangers of obesity.

Chapter 9

Exercise—a Fit Body for a Tireless Heart

D o you exercise? What is your routine? Taking a walk around the block in the evening? Spending some time on the Stairmaster? Swimming regularly? Playing tennis, basketball or racquetball?

Do people know about your exercise regimen? Is it regular enough that your friends think of it as a normal part of your life?

Exercise can do more for you than any pill on the market, any surgery offered by the best hospitals or any procedure done in a heart doctor's office. It is a surefire, no-miss, win-win situation for you and your heart, and it will keep you healthier than almost any other life change you can make.

Every person should have an exercise habit. One of the main causes of heart disease is the sedentary American lifestyle. The word *sedentary* comes from the same root as *sediment,* and the metaphor applies: Just as a river can get gummed up by dirt and debris, our arteries can, too. Most Americans subscribe to the sedentary lifestyle that has made our country famous. Yes, we are industrious, but we are also ingenious at finding ways to increase our leisure activity and decrease our physical activity with task-performing gadgets.

> Exercise can do more for you than any pill on the market, any surgery offered by the best hospitals or any procedure done in a heart doctor's office.

How often do you drive to the store or the post office, less than half a mile away, when a bike ride would be far more pleasant? Have you replaced your push mower with a riding mower? Have you hired neighborhood kids to do the trimming for you? How often do you take the elevator when the stairs are readily available?

Lack of exercise has clearly been shown to contribute to heart disease.[1] A quarter million deaths per year in the U.S.—about 12 percent of total deaths—are because of a lack of regular physical activity. A dismal one in five American adults gets enough exercise to help their hearts.

Studies also show that:

- At least half of youth do not engage in physical activity that promotes long-term health.
- Less than 36 percent of elementary and secondary schools offer daily physical education classes.
- Most classes were unlikely to foster lifelong physical activity.[2]

Exercise is like eating broccoli: Everybody knows it's good for you, but nobody wants to do it. And when reports come out that show that exercise reduces heart disease, they are treated as humdrum or "been-there, done-that." People know the truth, but they want an alternative—a drug, a new type of food, anything to let them retain their lifestyle.

Recently a major study was released that showed how a healthy lifestyle slashes the chance of heart disease by 82 percent.

Can you imagine! If a drug came out that did the same thing it would make headlines for weeks, and yet news reports of this study were limited to a few inches of text buried on the inside pages.

This landmark study, called the Nurses' Health Study, was conducted at the Harvard School of Public Health. It was the first to show what happens when people do everything they are supposed to—eat right, exercise, don't smoke, don't be overweight, drink moderately.

The study involved eighty-four thousand nurses—a pretty big group. Those who followed the rules of healthy living—including exercising vigorously for half an hour a day—reduced their risk of heart attacks, congestive heart failure and stroke by 82 percent compared with other women in the study.[3]

It says that the results "are very dramatic because these are not drastic changes for people. Premature heart disease can be virtually eliminated by these lifestyle changes."[4]

OVERWHELMING EVIDENCE

You can actually add years to your life by exercising regularly. If you start exercising at age thirty-five, studies show that you can add 6.2 months to your life. Imagine what you could do if you began even earlier![5]

What does it take to get you outside, in the gym or on the playing field? Nice weather? An invitation? Accountability to an exercise buddy? Surveys show that exercise is much more common in the "thin" states like Arizona and Colorado, where almost 15 percent of the population take bike rides or walk every day.[6] Some of the credit goes to the local governments who build bike lanes along new roads and widen the old ones to make room for exercisers. The beautiful scenery also draws people to spend more time outdoors.

> You can actually add years to your life by exercising regularly.

Do whatever it takes to get the heart pumping. Even walking in the evening will help. One study of retired men in Hawaii found that those who walked more than two miles per day had half the mortality rate of those who walked less than one mile per day.[7] This means that the men who walked the most lived five years longer than those who walked the least! That is good news for you. The power of lengthening life is in your hands.

IT'S ALL GOOD

The main thing to understand about exercise is that there is virtually no downside. While drugs to reduce cholesterol or suppress hunger have strange and perhaps unknown side effects, exercise is good for the whole person and can only help the body.

- It does not involve putting chemicals into our bodies.
- It lengthens our life span.
- It reduces our risk of heart disease.
- It can cure depression better than prescription drugs.
- It lowers blood pressure.
- It lowers body weight.
- It lowers the risk of developing diabetes.
- It lifts our spirits.
- It triggers other healthy lifestyle changes like improving our diet or quitting smoking.[8]
- It makes you look good.

Outside of infecting you with a measure of narcissism, the only possible disadvantage to exercise is that you might injure yourself somehow, but frankly, people who are out of shape and overweight are more at risk of injuring themselves in the course of everyday life. It is much easier for an overweight person to twist his or her ankle because of the extra weight on the leg, and it is probably more common for out-of-shape people to not respond as quickly when faced with a situation that demands quick action to prevent injury.

The good news is that exercise is becoming more popular. The bad news is, exercise isn't always accompanied by a healthy living strategy.

In Great Britain, health and fitness have become something of a craze in the past few years. A 1999 survey found that fitness and running were the UK's favorite exercise pastimes and that the fastest growing leisure sector was sporting goods and toys. The BBC called Britain's new fancy a national obsession with health.

147

> While drugs to reduce cholesterol or suppress hunger have strange and perhaps unknown side effects, exercise is good for the whole person and can only help the body.

But that healthy lifestyle only went so far. The same survey found that 29 percent of the population did not care what they ate as long as it tasted good![9]

Exercise, of course, should be paired with a host of lifestyle changes. I suggest that you integrate the new habits into your life as soon as you can, but at a reasonable pace. Do it as a family. If you have tried exercising only to peter out after a week or two, perhaps you need to make it a joint venture with your spouse, a relative or a friend. People are more likely to adopt heart-healthy habits if their partners do the same.

> It was found that persons who reduced their risk factors the most had a spouse who also significantly reduced his or her risk factors.[10]

Name your sport: Racquetball, tennis, swimming, jogging, aerobics classes—anything that gets the heart going every day for a half hour or more is beneficial. You might think you can't afford the time—and I agree. If you don't give up a half-hour every day now, you will lose potentially years later on.

Add quality and quantity to your life with regular exercise. I promise you, the difference it makes in every aspect of your life will be obvious.

Chapter 10

Quit Smoking
for Your Heart's Sake

I f exercise is one of the best things you can do for your heart,
smoking is one of the worst. Smoking cigarettes is like
putting a hole in your heart and letting the life leak out of it.
Few habits damage the heart more.

It's a shame that teen smoking is on the rise after several
decades of a steady decline in overall smoking. Society and
many state governments have taken strong stands against
tobacco, suing (and winning against) tobacco companies,
launching anti-smoking campaigns and legislating limits on
where people can smoke.

And yet, smoking is still with us, and our hearts are worse
off for it. Cigarettes consist of at least forty-three different
cancer-causing substances, plus thousands of others that are
capable of mutating our genes and poisoning our very bodies.

The damage to our lungs caused by smoking is well
known, but less well known is the damage it does to our
hearts and circulatory system. According to the American
Heart Association, as many as 30 percent of all heart disease

149

deaths in the United States each year are attributable to cigarette smoking. That is an amazingly large percentage. In effect they are saying that heart disease could be cut by a third if people would stop smoking.[1]

The Centers for Disease Control reports that, "During 1990, 418,690 U.S. deaths were attributed to smoking...A total of 179,820 of these deaths resulted from cardiovascular diseases."[2]

> Smoking literally steals days, weeks and years from people's lives.

The overall effect of cigarettes on the cardiovascular system is to increase general wear and tear while compromising the body's usual ability to function under duress. Smoking acts in combination with the other major risk factors—high blood pressure, high cholesterol, physical inactivity, obesity and diabetes—to compromise the body's cardiovascular health.[3]

Nicotine, tobacco's infamous ingredient, is known to harden arteries, cause blood clots and reduce the blood's capacity to deliver oxygen. Nicotine damages the cells lining the blood vessels and causes blood to stick to artery walls. Nicotine and other components of cigarette smoke greatly increase blood pressure and heart rate.[4]

Smoking even a single cigarette "appears to increase the coagulability of blood. The blood becomes stickier than the blood of nonsmokers," said Dr. Giri Saytendra of the University of Connecticut School of Medicine. "This means that clots are more likely to form and that the clots formed will be larger."[5]

How does smoking affect your chances of getting heart disease? Smoking a pack of cigarettes a day doubles your chances of having a heart attack. Smoking two or more packs a day triples the risk. A smoker is five times less likely to survive a heart attack than a nonsmoker, and someone who continues to smoke after having a heart attack will almost surely have another, more serious attack.[6]

Smoking literally steals days, weeks and years from people's lives. Men who smoke lose an average of eleven minutes of life for each cigarette. That means that eliminating one carton of cigarettes would buy the smoker an extra day and a half of life—enough time to fly round the world, take in a concert or enjoy a romantic night away.[7]

SECONDHAND SMOKE

Smoking harms the innocent. Children who are exposed to cigarette smoke have low levels of vitamin C in their blood regardless of how much vitamin C they obtained through food and multivitamins.

According to a report conducted by researchers at a major university, "Although intake of fruit, a major source of vitamin C, was similar among children with smoking and nonsmoking parents, blood levels of the vitamin were lower in children exposed to tobacco smoke. Vitamin C protects against metabolic changes that can lead to heart disease… [T]he report highlights the dangers of passive or second-hand smoke to children… Other studies have linked second-hand smoke to lower blood levels of vitamin C and beta-carotene in adults, and to an increased risk of asthma and wheezing in children."[8]

CIGARS

Cigarettes are not the only tobacco products to blame. Cigars appear to have the same ill effects. It used to be only older men who smoked cigars, but not anymore. Cigar smoking has risen 50 percent since 1993, especially among younger men and even women.

Cigars don't carry the warnings cigarettes do, and they have become a status symbol of types. Who hasn't seen copies of *Cigar Aficianado* month after month bearing pictures of Hollywood stars smoking their favorite cigar?

> Every time someone opens a pack of cigarettes he is playing Russian roulette, with more than one bullet, with his heart's future.

And yet cigars, the so-called "safe" alternative, increase the risk of heart disease. People who smoke more than four cigars a day are exposed to the equivalent of ten cigarettes a day. This is because the average smoker takes seven minutes to smoke a cigarette while most cigars take from sixty to ninety minutes.

For years, it was thought that because many cigar smokers do not inhale, they were exempt from the potential harm caused by the exposure. However, studies have shown that cigar smokers who do not inhale are still at risk.

The study found that "regular cigar smoking increases the risk of cardiopulmonary heart disease, chronic obstructive pulmonary disease, and cancers of the upper aerodigestive tract and lung. Individuals who smoke more than four cigars a day are exposed to an increased amount of smoke, the equivalent of ten cigarettes a day."[9]

Not only that, but cigars are unfiltered, meaning that the smoke from cigars has more nicotine, lead nitrogen oxides, ammonia, carbon monoxide and other devastating compounds than cigarettes.[10]

Cigar smokers also expose themselves to both the mainstream smoke from inhaling the unlit end of the cigar and the sidestream smoke from the burning end. Altogether, cigar smokers have a 68 percent higher risk of dying from lung cancer, heart disease or chronic obstructive lung disease than those who have never smoked.[11]

Why would a person choose to smoke when its harmful effects are so well known? I'm not sure, but every time someone opens a pack of cigarettes he is playing Russian roulette, with more than one bullet, with his heart's future.

The good news is that the damage can be reversed. "As soon as you stop smoking," says one medical authority, "your body begins to heal itself from the devastating effects of tobacco."[12]

Twenty minutes after you stop smoking, your blood pressure goes back down. Within a day your chance of a heart attack decreases, and by two months your circulation improves. After a year, your risk of heart attack is half what it would have been had you continued smoking, and after two years it is almost the same as the risk of a nonsmoker.[13]

Smoking robs us of energy, turns teeth yellow and makes breath smell bad. Smoking has even been found to promote gum disease.[14]

We will see in a later chapter why gum health is important to heart health.

Chapter 11

Don't Develop Diabetes or High Blood Pressure

I t has been a stressful day at work. You are up against impossible deadlines. Your head pounds, your eyes swim, and the voice of your boss echoes in your ears. "Get it done; I don't care what it takes…" The clock says 4 P.M., but you know the working day has just begun. You will be here through the night.

The phone rings. It's a client demanding to know what happened to his order. You buy some time with him, and the phone rings again. It's your boss requesting an immediate meeting in her office. You feel your heart race. Your whole body tightens up as you walk the hallway. "This has to be ruining my health," you mutter to a colleague.

"Just another day in the high blood pressure zone," he says, chuckling.

High blood pressure is one of the leading contributors to heart disease. It is caused by many different factors, including stress and smoking. As many as fifty million Americans have high blood pressure, and a third of them don't know it. But having our blood pressure checked regularly is one of the

155

best front-line defenses we have against hard arteries. Studies show that a person with high blood pressure can have twice the normal risk of heart disease.[1]

We all joke about certain situations, or even people, that drive up our blood pressure. What exactly do we mean? What is blood pressure, and what does it measure?

> High blood pressure is one of the leading contributors to heart disease. It is caused by many different factors, including stress and smoking.

Blood pressure is the amount of force that is exerted on the artery walls. Your blood pressure varies widely during a day, depending on your activity level. It is lowest while you are sleeping and highest while you are exercising. When you are frightened or in a stressful situation, hormones tell the heart to beat faster, which increases blood pressure temporarily.[2]

High blood pressure speeds up the process of hardening of the arteries. The increased pressure on the inner walls of blood vessels makes them more vulnerable to a buildup of fatty deposits.[3] And when arteries harden, they by definition lose elasticity, which drives blood pressure up even more.

The victim is the heart. High blood pressure forces the heart to work harder to keep blood flowing to the body. Think of when you blow up a balloon. Once the balloon has reached a certain point of elasticity, you have a more difficult time blowing air into it. Your lungs have to squeeze harder to push the air into the balloon.

That is how the heart responds to high blood pressure. When blood pressure is high for a long time, the heart grows larger, just as muscles in our arms or legs grow when we lift weights. The heart is actually "working out" to meet the extra demand. For a while the enlarged muscle has the strength to pump the blood against the high pressure, but then the large heart grows stiff and weak and becomes less effective than before.[4] This process may take years, and it leads to congestive heart failure and heart attacks.

The good news is that high blood pressure is easily detectable and usually controllable.[5] We have already discussed some of the things that bring on high blood pressure: smoking and an improper diet. The best advice, again, is to keep your arteries soft and elastic, not hard and encrusted, by eating right, taking supplements, exercising and not smoking. (We will talk about stress and attitude in a later chapter.) Your body will reward you for your effort.

DIABETES

Another major contributor to heart disease is diabetes, which is caused by lack of exercise, an unbalanced diet and obesity. Diabetes affects at least sixteen million Americans, putting them at much greater risk of heart disease than the general population.[6]

For example, women aged fifty-five with diabetes are seven times more likely to have heart disease than women without diabetes. In recent years, heart disease deaths for women with diabetes have actually increased while overall heart disease mortality for women has decreased.[7]

Diabetics are more likely to have their arteries clog up again after surgery to open them and are more likely to die following angioplasty. "[Re-clogging of the arteries] is one of the strongest predictors of (death after angioplasty) in the diabetic population," said the study. "This study indicates that diabetics should be treated differently from the general population."

> Diabetes affects at least sixteen million Americans, putting them at much greater risk of heart disease than the general population.

Why diabetics suffer more after heart surgeries is unclear, but doctors note that high levels of insulin in the blood can affect clotting and other systems that affect blood vessel walls.[8]

It is not known exactly why diabetes causes heart disease, but it may be that certain proteins that clear fat from the blood may not work as well in high blood sugar levels. This excess fat may block blood flow in the arteries.

"Clearance is the problem," said a researcher. "This excess fat may build up in the arteries of diabetics, making them more prone to atherosclerotic heart disease and a number of other complications of diabetes…[A]fter diabetics eat a meal, the fat in their blood tends to remain elevated longer than it does in people without diabetes."[9]

Diabetes is not a harmless disease. If you have it, consult your doctor about how to best combat it, or your heart may pay the price. If you don't have diabetes, don't develop it! There are ways to avoid it.

First, exercise! Type 2 diabetes (which affects 90–95 percent of people with diabetes) is linked to obesity and physical inactivity. According to the Centers for Disease Control, "Improving nutrition and increasing physical activity can delay the progression of diabetes."[10]

Exercise makes your muscles more sensitive to insulin, which improves the way your body metabolizes sugar.[11] Exercise will also keep your weight under control. Studies show that four out of five women with Type 2 diabetes are overweight.[13]

If you are a non-exerciser now, you need to turn the corner and become an active person. If you are overweight, this is especially important in light of the causes of diabetes. Losing weight will help your body use insulin better and will balance your blood sugar levels. Sometimes just ten or twenty pounds is enough to bring diabetes under control.[13]

And, of course, maintain a proper diet. This doesn't just mean laying off the sugar. Diabetes, because it is a disease involving blood sugar, was long thought to make people especially sensitive to eating table sugar and candy. Doctors and dietitians figured that simple sugars were more quickly digested and absorbed into the blood than complex carbohydrates, like the starch in potatoes and breads. They thought that table sugar would cause a larger rise in blood glucose and pose a threat to a diabetic person.

They were wrong. At least ten recent studies have shown that simple sugars don't spike blood glucose any higher or faster than other carbohydrates. The American Diabetes Association changed its nutritional recommendations in 1994. The new recommendations say, "Scientific evidence has shown that the use of sucrose as part of the meal plan does not impair blood glucose control in individuals with insulin-dependent (type I) or non-insulin-dependent (type II) diabetes."

The old guidelines that told you exactly how many teaspoons of sugar you could eat per week have been dropped.[14]

But that doesn't remove the dietary restrictions. It still isn't a good idea to eat refined sugar, or too much sugar of any kind, as we saw in an earlier chapter. The diet for preventing diabetes, and for controlling it when you have it, is the same as the diet for any other healthy person: Eat low-fat, balanced meals with plenty of fresh produce. Experts think that fruit and vegetable fiber help regulate blood sugar.[15]

Don't overeat, and don't load up on one kind of food.

If diabetes or high blood pressure are problems for you, consult your doctor and create a plan of escape so these conditions don't steal years from your heart.

Chapter 12

Don't Develop Gum Disease

You sit in the dentist's waiting room and wonder again why you let yourself get roped into another checkup. You hate everything about it: the terrible taste of the pumice scrub, the lectures about flossing, the fact that you have to keep your mouth open for a full twenty minutes and the inevitable discovery of new cavities.

Why see the dentist again? After all, you were just here...four years ago. Isn't that plenty often? You brush (usually), floss whenever there's a full moon and use that mouthwash (or is it really a breath freshener?).

Maybe your conscience got to you. Or maybe it was your spouse's nagging.

Just when you are eyeing the exit door, the dental assistant walks into the waiting room, plastic gloves on her hands, face mask pulled down around her neck. She looks at you and smiles—mischievously, it seems.

"Come on back. Haven't seen you for a while."

And you won't see me for another decade after this, you

161

think as you rise from your chair and march into the exam room like a man meeting his doom. You settle into the chair, which leans back too far—it always makes you tired—and there they are: the bright lights, the drills, the long, angular tools that will be used to prod, scrub and pick at your teeth. You sigh and accept the inevitable.

But what you don't know is that sitting in the dentist's chair might actually keep you from having a heart attack.

NEW FINDINGS

Obesity, smoking, diabetes, high blood pressure and lack of exercise are well-established causes of heart disease, but there are other causes as well that are just coming to light.

Every few years old ideas about heart disease get tossed out and new ones are born. Remember the days when people would talk about type A and type B personalities? It was commonly thought that different personalities were more prone to heart attacks, but that assumption has not fully explained why people have heart disease, and so you don't hear much about personality types anymore.

A doctor at Johns Hopkins University wrote, "The inability of 'traditional' risk factors such as [high cholesterol], [high blood pressure], and smoking to completely explain the incidence and trends in cardiovascular diseases has resulted in repeated calls for 'new risk factors.'"[1]

He means that the old ideas that high cholesterol and high blood pressure cause all heart disease are no longer valid. There are other factors, some mysterious, others just being discovered, that come into play.

Recent findings point the finger at a completely unsuspected foe: inflammation, most likely by a bacterial agent. More tests are showing a link between bacterial infection—such as the kind that causes gum disease—and heart disease. People with periodontal disease are one-third to more than two times more likely to have heart disease than people who do not have the condition.[2] That is a very strong relationship and suggests that bacteria may be a prime culprit in heart damage.

> Sitting in the dentist's chair might actually keep you from having a heart attack.

"Prevention of periodontal disease will likely reduce your risk of heart disease," says one leading researcher.[3]

The connection between mouth and heart is strong enough that the American Academy of Periodontology has issued a general health warning urging people who are at risk for heart disease or have signs of gum disease to consult a dentist. According to the Academy, "The AAP believes emerging research in this area may establish periodontal disease as a risk factor for cardiovascular disease...The Academy urges people who are at-risk for cardiovascular disease or have signs of gum disease to consult with a dentist experienced with treating periodontal disease."[4]

OLD IDEAS, NEW SUPPORT

The connection between oral health and heart health has long been known. In Germany, before doctors treat you, they send you to a dentist and take care of all your cavities and root canals, and they have shown much better results with cancer.

Doctors have known for decades that if some kinds of oral

bacteria enter the bloodstream during dental or heart surgery, they can cause "endocarditis," an often fatal heart infection. While this is rare, surgeons take great care to prevent it. Also, researchers have discovered that common viruses have been linked to heart disease.[5]

The human mouth is the body's biggest breeding ground of bacteria.[6] Half of American adults have gum disease.[7]

Oral bacteria enter the bloodstream through small ulcers in the gums. They are carried into the bloodstream and fought by the immune system. But some bacteria do not die, and they move throughout the body.

When those bacteria move from the mouth to the crown of the heart, they lodge in very small arteries and capillaries, which become inflamed, generate plaque and blood clots and kill the heart.[8]

Bacteria in the mouth have also been shown to make blood very sticky.[9]

Doctors have tested the effect of bacteria samples from patients with gum disease on human blood. In one test these bacteria were put in a test tube with human blood platelets, and the platelets began to clump together. This particular bacteria, which is the primary bacterial cause of adult gum disease, was the only bacteria to cause the platelets to clump. [10]

Studies also show that gum disease is a factor in strokes. One study found that bacteria from the mouth were in the hard, crusted artery walls of stroke victims.[11]

The problem goes back to diet and the tremendous amount of sugar and flour we consume, which gives us cavities and gum disease. Go to Africa and observe people who eat traditional foods and have no cavities, though they never brush their teeth!

The ancient Egyptians also suffered from horrible dental problems. Their diet was flour-based, as ours is, and it is entirely possible that the chronic infections they had in their gums and teeth led to heart disease, just as ours do.[12]

Today more doctors recognize that inflammation plays a role in heart disease. People who suffer from common chronic infections like infections of the sinuses, lungs or urinary tract are three times more likely to develop clogged arteries.[13]

> The human mouth is the body's biggest breeding ground of bacteria.

The idea of inflamed arteries does not rule out other causes of heart disease. It may be that inflammation and other causes work together and are to blame.

I believe that in the next few years, heart disease and plaque buildup will be treated with antibiotics—an idea that would have been heretical in the medical community a few years ago. There is still much to be learned about what causes the inflammations that harden arteries, but there are practical steps you can take right now.

FLOSS YOUR TROUBLES AWAY

One of my fundamental beliefs is that the body maintains a finely tuned biochemical balance, and that upsetting that balance causes a domino effect of health problems. No single illness or infection occurs in isolation.

When our teeth are constantly infected by periodontal disease, it is like having a wound that won't heal. Americans tend to brush for cosmetic reasons—to have whiter teeth or clean-smelling breath. But brushing and flossing are actually a first defense against heart disease and many other illnesses. Periodontal disease has been linked to diabetes, respiratory problems and premature births.[14]

The research shows that "gum disease may pose the greatest danger to your heart because the disease provides not only the bacteria, but also the conditions and opportunity for the bacteria to get into the blood through bleeding gums."[15]

What causes periodontal disease, and how can we get rid of it? I will leave a fuller answer of that question to your dentist, but I will note a few interesting facts I have discovered that may help you.

Vitamin C has been linked to a healthy mouth. People who eat less than the recommended daily allowance—60 milligrams—of vitamin C have higher rates of periodontal disease. This link has long been known. In the late eighteenth century, sailors away at sea would eat limes to prevent their gums from bleeding.[16]

If you needed another reason to take vitamin C supplements or eat a lot of citrus fruits, there it is!

Here is some general advice on what a healthy mouth looks like:

- Gums should be coral pink, not red, swollen or easy-to-bleed.
- Gums should fill the spaces between the teeth.
- Bacteria is reduced by brushing, flossing and rinsing with over-the-counter mouth washes.

It is all part of keeping that heart-healthy balance in our bodies—balance in our diet, in our level of physical activity, in our body weight, in our cleanliness habits.

If you are an occasional brusher, it's time to get regular about it. If you haven't flossed in a decade, it's time to dig the floss out of the back of your medicine drawer and put it to good use. The coming years will probably bring more confirmation that gum disease is a cause of heart disease, and when it does, you will be well ahead of the game.

Chapter 13

Detoxify Your Arteries With Chelation

Our Cardiac Research Institute at Oasis of Hope has all the technological advances, including a cath lab, and the newest technology, the "fast scan," which permits us to see coronary calcifications without invasive catheterization. Our cardiologists are experienced and renown in their specialty, but they are aware of the limitations of technology and the importance that lifestyle changes can achieve. Alternative treatments are researched and scientifically implemented.

After my father's diagnosis with life-threatening heart problems, he embarked on a series of lifestyle changes to help him beat the odds. He radically changed his diet, undertook a regular schedule of exercise, took supplements—and went through chelation therapy.[1]

We have talked about diet, exercise and supplements, and now I want to turn to the other aspect of my father's treatment that helped him overcome heart disease: chelation therapy.

Sometimes our arteries need to be swept clean of the

harmful substances that cause damage to the walls. Just as we take regular baths, our blood vessels should also be frequently washed to avoid heart disease. How do you do this? Many people, myself included, have embraced the benefits of a practice called chelation therapy.

Chelation means having a chemical solution injected into the arteries and given time to remove unwanted substances in the blood. The solution acts like a street sweeper, grabbing the trash and putting it away. The chemicals in the solution neutralize the harmful molecules that would otherwise damage our arteries. I and half a million other people each year have found that chelation produces tremendously positive results in our health and energy levels.

Chelation solution—the stuff that is put into the arteries—is a man-made amino acid called *ethylene diamine tetraacetic acid,* or EDTA. The word *chelation* comes from the Greek word for "claw," and that is what EDTA does: Binds to certain chemicals, metals or toxic substances and holds them like a stubborn crab. Not only is the toxic molecule held, it is incorporated into the structure of the EDTA so that it loses its toxicity altogether.[2]

The cardiologists in my father-in-law's hometown gave up on him. So he decided to come to Oasis of Hope for our heart-regenerating program, which includes diet, the supplements we have discussed earlier, close evaluation by our cardiologists (including management with whatever medications might improve quality of life) and other alternatives such as chelation therapy. He received forty chelation treatments and has now resumed all his normal activities, as well as started walking about two miles every day. He became a believer just as my father did!

TREATING LEAD POISONING

Where did this idea come from? Chelation has been used medically for years, though not for heart disease. In the 1940s and 1950s, chelation therapy was first employed in medicine to treat victims of lead poisoning, mostly sailors who had absorbed lead while painting ships. Chelation is still the treatment of choice for lead poisoning.[3]

> Just as we take regular baths, our blood vessels should also be frequently washed to avoid heart disease.

But the first time doctors realized chelation might have more wide-ranging benefits was when patients suffering both lead poisoning and hardening of the arteries reported surprising post-chelation improvements like less pain, more energy and more stamina. Doctors realized that just freeing the patients of lead was not bringing the results; it must be the treatment itself having an unknown benefit.[4]

They began to experiment with chelation on the worst, most incapacited heart disease sufferers and found that they improved. They had less pain, less shortness of breath, a normal body temperature in the extremities, better coordination and improved skin color. Many of these findings were published in scientific journals.[5]

One doctor wrote in a book about chelation, "The most promising treatment for premature aging of arteries, the most common form of which is atherosclerosis, is intravenous chelation therapy. This injection treatment apparently widens arteries that are narrowing and closing off blood flow. It reverses pathology [in]…a variety of malfunctions and disabilities where the basic issue is an interference with the flow of blood to a cell, tissue, organ or body part."[6]

> There are few risks involved with chelation. Patients usually drive themselves home after therapy and experience no side effects.

Many doctors through the years have recognized the value of chelation for patients suffering with hardened arteries, and yet heart patients are rarely told about chelation therapy before surgery or balloon angioplasty, although chelation is much safer at a fraction of the cost. Most insurance plans will not pay for it, and it is still considered controversial in the mainstream medical community.[7]

Some doctors say chelation is unproven, risky or in the least unhelpful in preventing heart disease. They argue that proper studies have not proven its benefit, and they dismiss the scientific basis for why chelation works. In response to testimonies of its effectiveness, they say the benefits came from other lifestyle choices like eating a proper diet, taking vitamin supplements and exercising.

The American Heart Association has said they find no scientific evidence to demonstrate any benefit from chelation therapy.[8]

But to me, the evidence clearly recommends chelation, and I am certainly not alone. Linus Pauling, the only person in history to receive two unshared Nobel prizes, was a chelation proponent. He wrote in 1988 that "EDTA chelation therapy fits in well with my views on healthcare...[It] is far safer and much less expensive than surgical treatments for atherosclerosis...[and] makes good sense to me as a chemist and medical researcher. It has a rational scientific basis, and the evidence for clinical benefit seems to be quite strong...Chelation has an equally valid rationale for use as a preventive treatment."[9]

On why doctors still reject chelation therapy out of hand, Pauling wrote, "Past harassment of chelating physicians by government agencies and conservative medical societies seems to stem largely from ignorance of the scientific literature and from professional bias."[10]

HOW TO GET
CHELATION THERAPY

There are an estimated fifteen hundred physicians in the U.S. who administer chelation therapy. The process begins with a complete examination and review of your medical history to make sure there are no allergies or existing medical conditions that would cause the therapy to somehow hurt you. Then you and the doctor decide on a schedule of infusions. Most people need twenty to fifty separate infusions. These are administered from one to five times per week until completed.[11]

The procedure takes place in the doctor's office—not in a hospital—and takes three to four hours. It requires you simply to sit and read a book, make phone calls, watch television, take a nap, chat with somebody or even catch up on your sewing while the chelating solution goes into your body via an intravenous needle. Some patients even run their business while being chelated![12]

There are few risks involved with chelation. Patients usually drive themselves home after therapy and experience no side effects. The risk of serious side effects, when chelation therapy is properly administered, is less than one in ten thousand patients treated. By comparison, the overall death rate as a direct result of bypass surgery is approximately three out of every hundred patients.[13]

Chelation therapy generally costs about $120 per treatment, or about $4,000 total. That is much less, of course, than the cost of bypass surgery or other procedures that would otherwise be required down the road.[14]

I recommend that people use chelation therapy preventively to rid their body of the harmful substances that inflame artery walls. It is a much-overlooked, but healthy approach to treating heart disease. For more information about chelation therapy, I have included a reading list at the back of this book.

IN CONCLUSION

I trust these keys to developing a healthy heart have been enlightening and helpful for you. Nevertheless, if a book about the heart addressed no more than properly caring for this wonderfully complex physical machine, it would be incomplete. For the heart is much more than a pump. Through time, the heart has been a metaphor for life, a symbol of the soul and a theme that transcends. The physical heart is inextricably connected with the soul, and to complete our look at this amazing organ, we must cast our gaze beyond the physical and examine the heart and soul.

SECTION III
HEART AND SOUL

Chapter 14

The Beat
Goes On

My nine-year-old daughter leaned her pretty head against my arm as I sat studying at my desk. Waving her completed homework in the air, she opened her mouth to speak. What came out astonished me.

"The right atrium *receives* blood from all the organs except the lungs through two large veins called the *superior vena cava* and inferior vena cava. It passes this oxygen-poor blood to the right ventricle, which then pumps the blood through the *pulmonary artery*. The pulmonary artery brings the blood to the lungs where it picks up oxygen from the air you breathe in.

"This oxygen-rich blood is returned to the left atrium of the heart by way of the *pulmonary veins*. This blood passes from the left atrium into the left ventricle to be pumped out to the rest of the body through the aorta.

"Amazing, isn't it?" she said, matter-of-factly tilting her head toward mine.

The description would have left me dizzy if I weren't a

medical doctor. But I had to agree that, indeed, the physiology of the heart is amazing. Even more amazing at that moment was that its functions had been so clearly stated by my nine-year-old daughter!

Still, I had to ask myself that although she grasped the mechanics of the heart, did she really understand the wonder of it? She knew it as a pump, but did she know it as the complex, intricate and enchanting organ that plays the drumbeat to every human life?

After twenty years of practicing medicine, did I understand the mysteries of the heart? Does any doctor fully grasp it?

Mysteries are a nuisance with which many people want to do away. Mysteries are responsible for superstitions and misguided beliefs. Science, we are told, exposes error and reveals truth.

How well I remember my first day of medical school when a professor told the class, "There are no mysteries in the human body that anatomy, physiology, molecular biology and pathology cannot explain."

No doubt he truly believed this. But for most of history, the heart was a tightly sealed mystery, and in some ways it remains so today.

THE ANCIENT HEART

You can probably point out the approximate location of your kidneys, liver, lungs, intestines and so on, but for most people throughout history, knowledge was only skin-deep. It is difficult for a modern person like you or me to imagine how little was known about the heart and the human body even a few hundred years ago.

Picture growing up without ever knowing exactly what was

underneath your skin. For centuries dissection was illegal.

There were no diagrams of the human body, no textbooks, no plastic models of human organs, no x-rays, no websites, no (accurate) medical books. Virtually no medical knowledge as we know it today existed at all. The only place someone might see the inside of the human body was on the battlefield or at the scene of a very unfortunate accident.

Nevertheless, even then people knew that the heart was very special. The slaughter and consumption of animals gave people familiarity with internal organs and showed them the heart's critical role in sustaining life. Cave drawings in Spain dating back thousands of years depict woolly mammoths with red hearts drawn on their chests, indicating where hunters should aim their spears.

Homer, the ancient Greek writer, described the death of a warrior in the *Iliad*, saying, "And he fell with a thud, and the spear was fixed in his heart, that still beating made the butt thereof quiver, till mighty Ares snuffed its fury out."[1]

> Although she grasped the mechanics of the heart, did she really understand the wonder of it? She knew it as a pump, but did she know it as the complex, intricate and enchanting organ that plays the drumbeat to every human life?

LIGHTER THAN A FEATHER

Through most of history, erroneous theories about the heart

179

and body abounded. Refuting them brought scorn from both religious leaders and enlightened men.

Clay tablets from the Babylonian empire in 4000 B.C. list sixty-two human malformations and their purported meanings, one of them being that "when a woman gives birth to an infant…that has the heart open and that has no skin over it, the country will suffer from calamities."[2]

The Aztecs offered sacrifices to their gods, but none were as important as the sun god. They believed that the sun would stop moving if they didn't offer it human hearts. No other organ would do.

The hearts of prisoners could appease the sun god for a day-to-day offering, but for special occasions, virgins and other members of the high society considered it an honor to give their hearts for such a holy purpose. Today's surgeons would be very impressed with the Aztecs' knowledge of anatomy and their extraordinary skill to extricate the heart in a blink of an eye.[3]

When the Egyptians embalmed someone, all organs were removed and placed in jars to be buried with the corpse—except for the heart, which remained with the body. According to their religion, deceased people entered the netherworld, and immediately their hearts, representing conscience and character, were weighed on a scale against a feather, representing truth and order. If the heart weighed less than the feather, the person was allowed into the afterlife.[4]

The Bible is filled with references to the heart. In the Book of Genesis, God looked upon the earth before He unleashed the flood and saw "that the wickedness of man was great in the earth, and that every imagination of the thoughts of his heart was only evil continually" (Gen. 6:5, KJV).

The Book of Proverbs says, "Let not mercy and truth forsake thee: bind them about thy neck; write them upon the table of thine heart" (Prov. 3:3, KJV). And again, "A sound heart is the life of the flesh: but envy the rottenness of the bones" (Prov. 14:30, KJV).

Indeed, the word *heart* appears in some 858 times in the King James Version of the Bible.[5] Throughout the Bible, the heart is considered in need of being:

- Cleansed
- Known by God
- Changed from stone to flesh
- Tried
- Circumcised
- Searched
- Sifted
- Written upon by the Holy Spirit
- Filled with God's words
- Washed
- Kept unafraid
- Kept untroubled
- Enlarged by love
- Made into a dwelling place for Christ

EDUCATED GUESSES

Aristotle, perhaps the most influential philosopher and thinker until the Renaissance, believed that the heart was the source of our thoughts and intelligence, a position reserved for the brain today. He also believed the heart was the seat of the soul.

Hippocrates—whose oath "Do no harm" has made him

one of the most famous physicians of all time—also believed that the heart was the seat of the intellect. He said it contained "human intelligence, the principle which rules over the rest of the soul."[6]

> Today's surgeons would be very impressed with the Aztecs' knowledge of anatomy and their extraordinary skill to extricate the heart in a blink of an eye.

Plato, Aristotle's teacher, believed that the heart, which he called "the knot of the veins and the fountain of the blood," was the abode of the passions. He considered them "terrible and irresistible affections" such as pleasure, pain, fear, anger and love. When these passions were aroused, according to Plato, the heart would beat faster and become inflamed and irrational until the lungs—which he associated with logic—intervened and "cooled" down the heart so that reason could prevail.[7]

Clearly, the heart has always been understood as having great importance, but for thousands of years nobody knew how it worked. Even learned men had few answers for the many questions posed by the heart and circulatory system. Obviously thumpings and bumpings were going on beneath the surface of the skin; when the flesh was cut, it bled, sometimes profusely. Still, the idea that the heart was a pump that sent blood through tiny "aqueducts" was completely unknown.

Ancient Egyptians believed that the heart and other major organs floated freely around the inside of the body of their own volition.[8] They also believed that most diseases were caused when fecal matter backed up in the bowels and made its way to the heart, resulting in infections, poor teeth and slow-healing wounds. To prevent this buildup they would give themselves enemas, and even pack the rectum with honey.[9]

As we already saw, they weren't so far off in their assessment of what caused the heart to become ill.

Aristotle did not grasp the fundamentals of the circulatory system or the heart's role in it. In his treatise *About the Movement of Animals,* he wrote that human movement was made possible by breath passing through the heart. In other words, he thought that when we breathed, air went into the heart and enabled us to move.

Aristotle is also credited with the earliest observations of heart function by describing the fetal pulsation in a chick embryo.

One Greek man, Alcmaeon of Croton (circa 500 B.C.), said that sleep was caused by blood draining from the brain via the veins. Death resulted when the brain completely drained of blood (which would technically be true, since the brain cannot survive long without the oxygen blood brings).[10]

Indeed, many of the ancients agreed that the heart was the body's source of heat. Hippocrates also believed that the heart and lungs acted as hot and cold counterbalances to each other.[11] He even recorded the symptoms of a heart attack in very modern terms. He said, "Sharp pains irradiating soon toward the clavicle and back are fatal."[12]

It may sound silly now, even to my daughter, but when you take into account that these theories came about through observations limited to placing a hand on their chests, breathing in and out and feeling a heartbeat, they actually make a lot of sense. I doubt that any of us could think of a better theory without the help of medical science.

SMALL STEPS TOWARD THE TRUTH

Over the years, truth advanced one small step at a time. But you can imagine how difficult it was to put all the pieces together. The pulse, for example, was not understood. Observers did not see a difference between a pulse and other movements that take place in the muscles, such as spasms or tremors. Herophilus of Chalcedon (280 B.C.) was the first to see the pulse as an indicator of health or disease. He studied its rate and rhythm and realized that the pulse was derived from the heart and was not merely a function of the arteries.

> Clearly, the heart has always been understood as having great importance, but for thousands of years nobody knew how it worked.

Another Greek observer, Erasistratos of Iulis (250 B.C.), developed Aristotle's theory about air passing through the heart. He said that air breathed into the lungs first passed to the left side of the heart and then to the arteries of the body. He believed that the arteries carried only air! Naturally, he also believed that the air passing through the arteries caused the heartbeat.

This view prevailed for almost four centuries until Claudius Galenus (A.D. 129–201) demonstrated that arteries carried blood and not air. He studied the actions of the heart, the heart valves and the pulsation of arteries, noting the structural differences between arteries and veins. Still, he didn't understand that blood circulated through the body. He believed that the liver produced blood and sent it to the body to form flesh.

Galen did not see the heart as the organ of intelligence. He demonstrated that compressing the brain caused loss of movement and thought processes, while compressing the heart only stopped the pulse.[13] In an experiment on a living pig, he severed the vocal cords to prove that ability to speak comes from the brain, not the heart. The pig's squeals instantly became nothing more than a whisper, and Galen noted that the nerves leading to the vocal cords led to the brain and not to the heart.[14]

He also believed that life was sustained by food, which he believed was converted into blood by the liver and sent to the rest of the body to nourish it. Blood was used in the removal of wastes as well, according to Galen, who was first to suggest a relationship between food, blood and air.

Galen also believed the heart was the body's "heater"; he called it "the hearthstone and source of the innate heat."[15] Medical and church authorities considered Galen's work to be divinely inspired and therefore infallible. Therefore, they dubbed him *Divinus Galenus*.

THE MANLY HEART

To many of the major figures in medical history, the heart and lungs seemed to reflect the relationship between male and female. The heart was entirely masculine: the source of heat, movement and even the source of reproductive capacity (some thought the heart was the source of sperm).[16] When

185

a person was enraged or smitten with love, it was the heart that responded passionately, beating with fury and causing the chest to turn red.

The lungs, on the other hand, were depicted in female terms. They were cool, moist, delicate, passive and embraced the heart to moderate its heat. The lungs did not seem to move of their own accord and were thin and spongy, instead of being thick and muscular like the heart.[17]

THE MERRY-GO-ROUND OF SCIENCE AND PHILOSOPHY

Scientific hypothesis and theories are constantly changing in our time, but in the Dark Ages, Galen's theories were dogma. For about eleven hundred years after Galen, very little was learned about the heart or any other part of the human body. Still, the mystery and mystique that surrounded the heart remained. One of England's most famous kings, Richard, was named "Lion Heart" because of his military prowess and reputation for chivalry. He became a central figure in English romance.[18]

POETRY OF THE HEART

The heart also thrived in literature of the Middle Ages. In Dante's classic *Inferno,* he wrote, "Consternation pierced my heart," and later that:

> The ice about thy heart melts as the snow
> On mountain heights, and in swift overflow
> Comes gushing from thy lips in sobs of shame.[19]

Indeed, the heart was also seen as the main gatekeeper to the soul, and its openness to the gospel was usually measured in terms of hot or cold. Anatomist Thomas Watson, who took a keen interest in the spiritual aspect of the heart, instructed people to "prepare your hearts for the reading of the Word. Leave not off reading in the Bible till you find your hearts warmed…Let it not only inform you, but inflame you…Go not from the Word till you can say as those disciples, 'Did not our heart burn within us.'"[20]

DEBUNKING THE MYTHS

But knowledge of the heart was confined to the poetic and religious realm until the Renaissance, when the practice of secret dissection led to rapid advances in knowledge as science began to debunk heart myths.

In 1513, artist and scientist Leonardo da Vinci (1452–1519) drew and described a defect he observed in a human heart.

In 1543, Andreas Vesalius (1514–1564) proposed that the heart was the center of the vascular network and that the pulmonary veins carried air from the lungs to the left atrium. Several other physicians demonstrated the relationship between the lungs and heart, and one physician discovered that veins have valves to keep blood from flowing backward.

Helkiah Crooke, an early modern anatomist, put the heart at the head of the royal court of critical body parts, which included the brain and liver. The heart, he said, was the king; the brain was the judge or governor, and the liver was the prince. "By his perpetual motion, all things are exhilarated and do flourish; and nothing in the whole creature is fruitful unless the powerful vigor of the heart gives it fecundity," he wrote.[21]

THE DISCOVERY OF CIRCULATION

But it was the English physician William Harvey (1578–1657) who finally shed light on the system of blood circulation. The first "cardiac biomechanist," Harvey was greatly influenced by Aristotle's theory of the primacy of the heart. He was the first to show the heart as the pump that pushed blood through the vascular system. This was a major advancement in understanding how the heart worked.[22]

Harvey showed the function of valves in maintaining flow in veins, establishing the concept of a circulation propelled by the heart and refuting the hallowed theories of Galen. Harvey also proposed the existence of capillaries, which link arteries and veins.[23]

THE MYSTIQUE REMAINS

The efforts to debunk "magical" practices and develop scientific methods for better diagnosis and treatment picked up speed. It was all part of the Enlightenment Age, a way of thinking that continues to dominate Western culture and our own American medical practices. The heart was correctly identified as a pump that pushed blood through the body via arteries, capillaries and veins. The theories of Aristotle and Galen, though clever, were laid aside in favor of empirical research. Suddenly the heart came under the rather unpoetic lights of clinical observation.

Nevertheless, in Shakespeare's time, even though there was quite a bit of scientific knowledge of the heart's anatomy, the heart never lost its mystical connotation. Throughout literature it is heralded as the seat of the human soul.

- From *Hamlet:* "In my heart's core, ay, in my heart of heart."
- From *Julius Caesar:* "Thy heart is big, get thee apart and weep."

ꙮ From *King Lear:* "O, madam, my old heart is crack'd, it's crack'd!"

But science is no longer fumbling in the dark. The twentieth century heralded the most comprehensive and astonishing advances in the understanding and treatment of the heart. But it is also important to realize that, despite an incredible increase of knowledge and technological know-how, the human heart remains one of the most enduring, powerful and mysterious symbols in our culture.

The heart is like Darwinism, in a way, in that its mystery endures in the face of plenty of scientific preaching. In spite of the massive indoctrination, "including a pitch for evolution on every public television program that deals with nature," says Phillip E. Johnson, "the state of public opinion hasn't changed in the last thirty years. Polls show that fewer than 10 percent of the American public

> Knowledge of the heart was confined to the poetic and religious realm until the Renaissance, when the practice of secret dissection led to rapid advances in knowledge as science began to debunk heart myths.

believes in the official scientific orthodoxy, which is that humans (and other living things) were created by a materialistic evolutionary process in which God played no role."[24]

189
ꙮ

In the same way, scientific knowledge and our emotional attachment to the heart now exist side by side. The unprecedented scientific knowledge we have has not stripped away the meaning we attach to this amazing muscle. If it is just a pump, why does our "heart" ache? And really, how do we mend a broken heart?

> Despite an incredible increase of knowledge and technological know-how, the human heart remains one of the most enduring, powerful and mysterious symbols in our culture.

Musicians from Mozart to the Beatles to N Sync all side with the mystical Aristotelian and biblical concept of the heart—despite the overwhelming scientific evidence that it is nothing more than a sophisticated piece of plumbing!

LANGUAGE OF THE HEART

The heart remains the most poetic, symbolic organ in our body. We speak of the heart in ways we would never speak of our gallbladder, our liver or even our sex organs. We wouldn't say, "I mean this from the bottom of my liver" or "My kidneys are overflowing with gratitude," because we see our other organs as physical entities. But our relationship with our own heart is much richer than that.

We say things like, "I mean this from the heart." "That guy is all heart." "You are tugging at my heart strings."

Literature, especially romantic literature, uses the heart to symbolize our most tender, vulnerable selves. Every February America is awash in red and pink hearts, symbolizing romance and love. We even put bumper stickers on our cars that say, "I [heart symbol] my dog."

The heart is not only the seat of our affections and our emotions, but it is also the very core of who we are. The heart is also the seat of our spirituality. All religious writings, especially the Bible, refer to the heart as the seat of life and our spirit. Jesus spoke about it often:

> Blessed are the pure in heart, for they will see God.
> —MATTHEW 5:8, NIV

He pictured the heart as a storehouse or safe where we keep our most important things:

> For where your treasure is, there your heart will be also.
> —MATTHEW 6:21, NIV

Jesus even described His own heart:

> Take my yoke upon you and learn from me, for I am gentle and humble in heart, and you will find rest for your souls.
> —MATTHEW 11:29, NIV

Jesus clearly saw the heart as the central decision-making organ, the place where we keep what is most dear to us. When asked, "What is the greatest commandment?", Jesus replied, "Love the Lord your God with all your heart and with all your soul and with all your mind" (Matt. 22:37, NIV).

The most eloquent anatomist cannot describe the beauty

within the skin of a fellow human. As a surgeon, I have experienced this most wondrous and beautiful of Creation's art many times, and the fascination has not abated. Understanding the heart's function and biology has not demystified it for me. Knowing how it works does not answer the most important and ultimate question: Why?

> The heart is not only the seat of our affections and our emotions, but it is also the very core of who we are.

Why our heart aches, suffers, overflows and rejoices is a question probably best answered by poets, priests and philosophers. Still, doctors can certainly learn this: The heart and its health is much more complex than our research has yet told us.

Nevertheless, the heart, even with all its mysteries, really is a pump. Granted, it is a marvel of a pump, but thanks to many dedicated scientists we now understand it, at least physiologically. Its complexity is masterfully managed by simple laws of physics. These, when observed, will pave the heart's path for a long and smooth journey. The better you care for your heart, the longer it will care for you.

Chapter 15

Take Heart

I t wasn't science fiction. There were no lightning bolts, eerie assistants or mad white-coated scientists with frenzied hair and wild eyes. Nevertheless, it was a strange human experiment. In 1984, scientists transplanted the heart of a baboon into a twelve-day-old baby girl, known as Baby Fae.

A team of medical scientists from Loma Linda University in California performed the operation. Although Baby Fae died twenty-one days later, the experiment contended that the human experiment provided valuable research information for the future.[1]

If a human heart were nothing more than a muscle pump, then any pump would do, even that of a monkey or a pig. And if humans are merely highly evolved apes, then why not? But intrinsic wisdom tells us that much more is involved. And if the human heart is the seat of the soul, is it also what makes us truly human? If so, then this "valuable" research was extracted at a terrible cost to a tiny, defenseless human being.

WHERE THE HEART RESIDES

For centuries, scientists, doctors and philosophers have debated the location of the soul. For centuries it was thought that the soul was located in the heart muscle itself. Then the belief shifted, and the soul was thought to reside in the brain. Increasingly, doctors don't believe in the soul as a spiritual entity anymore, but they are very interested in finding the mythical "heart" that makes up our emotions, consciousness and perceptions of the world.

New findings in the fields of behavioral genetics and cognitive neuroscience are building a bridge between the long-separated fields of science and the arts. Scientists are realizing that such things as love, morality and appreciation of beauty originate in the brain and can be treated as physical phenomenon. A fundamental division between the humanities and sciences may become as obsolete as the division between the celestial and terrestrial spheres.[2]

With all of this searching, will a person's soul, his true heart, prove to be simply an illusion? Some experimenters think so. A man named Kevin Warwick has been trying to harness the power of human thoughts and turn the brain into a useful machine. He literally wants computers to learn to read human minds, making "electronic telepathy" the new mode of communication. People could "think" to one another rather than talk. Information could be downloaded directly into the brain.[3]

To Warwick, the human heart and its habits are outmoded and slow. Turning thoughts into intelligible language takes too much time. Instead, he says, we can train computers to read electrochemical signals in our body and brain (transmitted by an implant in a person's body) and eventually communicate with people in the same way.

But what happens to the individual heart and soul when all of our brains are linked together? Does it devalue our individuality? Our emotions? Our deeply held feelings and beliefs?

Not all scientists want to get rid of the soul. In recent years, some scientists have actually claimed that the "soul" will soon be found. Susan Greenfield, leading researcher and professor of synaptic pharmacology at the University of Oxford, has been tackling that problem for years. Her goal is to find the seat of the soul—the true "heart" of humanity—by discovering how wildly complex chemicals in the brain generate a sense of consciousness. If she can pin down which areas of the brain and which chemicals are involved in certain reactions—like the sense of well-being we get from seeing a flower garden or smelling freshly brewed coffee—she thinks she can solve the puzzle of human consciousness and, in a sense, isolate the human soul.

> Scientists are realizing that such things as love, morality and appreciation of beauty originate in the brain and can be treated as physical phenomenon.

Greenfield's theory is that consciousness emerges from the activity of groups of nerve cells in the brain. In her book, *Journey to the Centers of the Mind,* she writes: "The more I heard, read and thought about it, the more it seemed incredible that mere molecules could in some way constitute an inner vision, idea or emotion, or—even more astounding—

that they could generate the subjectivity of an emotion. Yet consciousness is continuous with the brain's activity and must emerge from it."[4]

She and other scientists have begun using high-powered brain scanners to produce a picture showing which parts of the brain are used for different tasks. And yet Greenfield remains pessimistic about actually finding the soul—the true heart of a human being.

"I don't think the problem of consciousness will be solved," she says. "Just because [other theories are outdated] does not mean that we will be able to solve the hard problem of consciousness."

I agree that efforts to find the mythical "heart" among so many chemicals and brain cells will ultimately fail. Scientists will find that chemical reactions do cause emotions, mind-sets, personalities and habits, but they will be no closer to finding the "heart and soul" of a person than when they began because a person's true heart is spiritual and eternal. It cannot be summed up by a combination of chemicals or pinned down to a laboratory table.

A WINNING ATTITUDE

Your real heart—the one we refer to poetically and philosophically—is the most important part of your being. It gives spiritual life and sustenance and can be the reservoir for love and goodwill, or a well of anger and resentment. In it we hide our deepest thoughts and feelings.

So we have, whether we want to or not, to deal with many hearts: the incredibly awesome pump that gives physical life, the emotional, the spiritual, the learning, and so on, and the "real" heart, the one that gives meaning to a life that does not end with death. This heart I'll call the "transcendent heart."

Even in this aspect of transcending the physical, the biblical codes are applicable to all. You may strip the religious and spiritual aspects and benefit from the emotional and meditative benefits it will bring to the physical heart, but the Bible is unique also in this field, and if you want, you can reap a lot more than just physical health.

Our transcendent heart holds the things we cherish and becomes like a private room that we only open up for those we trust the most. The heart is where man meets God, where God speaks to man and where our human nature reconciles itself with the divine.

Not only that, but this transcendent heart will go on forever. It does not die with the rest of our body. It does not

> A person's true heart is spiritual and eternal. It cannot be summed up by a combination of chemicals or pinned down to a laboratory table.

cease when the chemicals stop flowing in our brains. It is something outside the realm of scientific study and bizarre experimentation. It goes beyond biological theories. Instinctively we know this, though we have been trained to look to scientists for all the answers.

We know that the transcendent heart exists because that is where the important aspects of our lives take place. And we know that from this transcendent heart springs health or sickness, depending on what shape our spiritual heart is in.

THE HEART:
THE CROSSROADS OF HEALTH

Increasingly, doctors are coping with the fact that the physical heart muscle is impacted by our eternal transcendent heart's health. Happiness, sadness, love and anger all contribute positively or negatively to the well-being of our heart muscle.

> When it comes to heart health, our perceptions, emotions and attitudes can save us or kill us.

Recall a time when you were "falling in love." Was there not an unexplainable "melting" in your chest when you saw your beloved? Or, if you think about someone you have loved deeply—a parent, child or friend—do you not feel a warm sensation in your chest? And what about negative emotions such as anger, anxiety and fear? There is a growing body of evidence to support the concept that what you feel in your eternal heart does affect what you feel. And whatever a person feels affects the heart muscle at its most fundamental level.

A friend and I were skiing in Colorado one time when he took a path down the mountain that he shouldn't have. He crashed into a tree and was suddenly in tremendous pain. I knew that he at least had fractured a few ribs. He had great difficulty breathing. The paramedics arrived promptly, immobilized him and installed a heart monitor to make sure his heart was not affected. Though his pain was excruciating, he was not in danger of losing his life.

Soon after our arrival at the emergency clinic the doctor came in. She was young and strikingly beautiful. As she began to examine my friend, I noticed that his monitor started almost rattling with tachycardia (rapid heartbeat) and that his blood pressure increased. The pained look on his face disappeared, and he appeared as comfortable and relaxed as if he were sitting in a spa. She installed a bandage all around his chest, normally a painful procedure, but he never complained. As soon as she left the room he exhaled audibly, "I'm in love." His rapid heartbeat and pain were overshadowed by the pleasurable sensations of excitement and passion. Instead of tachycardia he felt "heart flutters" and actually felt exuberant and "lighthearted."

That is one example of how our emotional heart can affect our physical heart. Perception has a lot to do with how we interpret, consciously or unconsciously, what may be going on in our hearts.

And when it comes to heart health, our perceptions, emotions and attitudes can save us or kill us.

FEAR

I remember the first time I measured the blood pressure of a patient who came for a routine physical. She was completely calm as I began the procedure. But as I fumbled with the cuff and made obvious my inexperience, she began to experience palpitations—a sensation of pounding, irregularity of the heartbeat—and the pressure gauge went through the roof. As much as I wanted to relate her reaction to my youth and good looks, I knew that it was something else: She was terrified!

Emotions such as fear and panic can trigger an adrenaline "rush" that overstimulates your heart, your increasing heart rate often out of sync by the addition of extra beats. As you feel your heart speeding up or beating irregularly, you become even more anxious, prompting your system to pump out even more stress hormones—and the vicious cycle continues.

All of this is to say that our emotions, attitude and even personality can directly affect our heart health.

ANGER

The Bible says that out of the overflow of the heart, the mouth speaks. It is safe to say that whatever is in a person's spiritual heart will spill over into his or her life in a variety of ways. Take anger, for example. Heart disease used to be considered more common in people with type-A personalities—people who were competitive, perfectionist, impatient and prone to hostility. Now only type-H personalities—people who are overly hostile—are believed to have higher risk for heart disease. A survey found that people who scored high on the hostility scale were seven times as likely to die by age fifty compared to their peers, and the difference was largely due to increased incidence of heart disease.[5]

Angry responses cause wear and tear on the whole body, including the cardiovascular and immune systems.

This can be explained physiologically: When you are angry, a "fight-or-flight" response is engaged in the brain, and the hormone noradrenalin is released directly into the heart, causing it to beat up to five times harder than normal. The diameter of blood vessels throughout the body decreases, forcing blood into muscles and raising blood pressure dramatically. Not only that, but when you are angry, fat is released into the bloodstream.[6]

See how the eternal heart impacts the physical heart? It isn't possible to keep those emotions bottled up inside of you. Like a poison, they leak into your very bloodstream and damage the heart pump.

Are you an angry person? Do small things get on your nerves? Do you fly off the handle more than you should? It might not be just a character flaw—it may be taking years off your life.

STRESS

Stress has a similar effect as anger, causing arteries to constrict and the heart to work harder. Stress is like having an angry reaction at a subdued level over a long period of time.

Stress responses are actually good for us—in some cases. They give us a temporary boost of strength and freedom from pain. You have probably heard of people who performed superhuman feats, such as lifting a car off a child. What happens in those instances is that the sympathetic nervous system (SNS) has kicked in, releasing hormones like adrenaline and norepinephrine. This release of physical power, negation of pain and mobilization of energy can actually save your life.

But chronic activation of your SNS from daily stressors has tremendous potential to harm you for two reasons. The first is wear and tear on your heart and circulation. The second happens when body systems shut down to fuel states of hyperarousal. Digestion, immune system activity, sexual drive and repair of tissues are all inhibited. In fact, research has shown that staying in SNS "overdrive" increases your risk of developing one form of diabetes, and there is evidence that stress-induced high blood pressure can encourage the formation of atherosclerotic plaques.

One doctor observed at the end of the Vietnam War that a

lot of ostensibly healthy young people were having heart attacks. They were reacting to the stress of losing their jobs because of all the defense cutbacks. He saw unemployed defense workers as young as twenty-nine dropping dead from worry.

Doctors "must understand that disease is not just a physical event," he said. "I can't think of one illness that does not have a psychological/emotional as well as spiritual component."[7]

> A problem in our emotional heart directly affects our physical heart.

People who have a hard time dealing with financial strain develop gum disease more often than those who handle it well, one study has shown. Doctors postulated that people who don't deal well with money stress are more apt to grind their teeth, skip brushing and flossing and experience a weakening of the body's ability to fight infection. It is conceivable that money strain or stress of any kind can lead to heart disease by lowering our immune abilities and prompting gum disease.[8]

Stress is an enemy of the heart, whatever form it comes in.

DEPRESSION

Some people's spiritual hearts fill up with great sadness or depression. Depression has been linked to an increased risk of coronary disease. A study published in the July 1998 issue of *Archives of Internal Medicine* revealed that men who had experienced an episode of major depression had twice the risk of developing heart disease.

A 1996 study reported in *Circulation*, an official journal of the American Heart Association, that people who had a two-week mild depression also had twice the risk of heart disease; a history of more serious depression quadrupled the risk. Another *Circulation* study showed up to a 70 percent higher risk for heart disease in depressed people.

Depression affects the way your nervous system regulates your heart rate and blood vessel activity. Depressed people tend to have faster heart rates, higher blood pressure and "stickier" platelets (clotting components) in their blood.[9] Depression may also increase mental stress, which in turn encourages blockage of the blood vessels.

Statistics show that as many as 30 percent of people sixty-five and older are depressed, yet only 1 percent receive treatment.[10]

Again, a problem in our emotional heart directly affects our physical heart.

BYE-BYE BLUES

Conversely, exercising our physical heart muscle can have a wonderful effect on the spiritual heart. Recently a study was conducted that involved one hundred fifty-six people suffering from depression. The group was divided into three groups.

- One group was given antidepressants only.
- One group was given antidepressants plus group aerobics (thirty minutes three times a week).
- One group was not given antidepressants but was put on an exercise regimen.

After nine months, only 30 percent of those in the exercise-only group were still depressed, while more than half of the people in the other groups were depressed.

Doing only fifty minutes of exercise a week has been shown to cut your chances of being depressed in half. Many studies show cognitive behavioral therapy can be as effective as drugs.[11]

A HEALTHY
MARRIAGE HELPS THE HEART

Loving relationships, especially long-lasting marriages, help the spiritual and physical hearts immensely.

> Just as the Bible was ahead of its time in identifying a healthy diet, so it also holds the key to a healthy heart, both physically and spiritually.

In a study of nearly five hundred middle-aged women, researchers at the University of Pittsburgh in Pennsylvania found that marital distress was linked to a higher risk for heart problems.

This study, which followed the women over a period of about eleven years, was an attempt to gauge how marital satisfaction affects heart health as women go through menopause. Women who reported marital dissatisfaction were more likely than satisfied women to have significant plaque buildup in the main artery of the heart. They were also more likely to have blockages in the carotid arteries in the neck, a known risk factor for stroke.

Unhappiness in a marriage may harm the heart by inflicting "wear and tear" on the body, said one of the study's authors. Like stress in general, marital dissatisfaction may lead to habitual elevations in heart rate, blood pressure and stress hormones.[12]

In his book *Love & Survival* (HarperCollins, 1998), Dean Ornish wrote, "I am not aware of any other factor in medicine—not diet, not smoking, not exercise, not stress, not genetics, not drugs, not surgery—that has a greater impact on our quality of life, incidence of illness and premature death from all causes."[13]

FEAR NOT

Just as the Bible was ahead of its time in identifying a healthy diet, so it also holds the key to a healthy heart, both physically and spiritually. Proverbs 4:4, 23 says, "Lay hold of my words with all your heart; keep my commands and you will live...Above all else, guard your heart, for it is the wellspring of life" (NIV).

Many people are overcome by fear, anger and sadness. They are afraid of death because they do not know where they will go once their heart stops beating. They are angry because they have not found their life's purpose. They are sad because they have not found the source of love. All these things affect the physical heart—and the spiritual heart, the one that goes forever.

There are many ways of finding relaxation and controlling harmful emotions. Stress-management techniques, long vacations, even depression-fighting drugs can improve life for many people.

But none of these can solve the central questions that every person asks. Only Jesus Christ can take away our fear of death, can give us a purpose, can become that wellspring of life and love that we long for.

God so loved the world that He gave His only Son so that you and I could have everlasting life. (See John 3:16.) That kind of news makes my physical heart leap and my spiritual heart soar!

Accepting Christ can do wonders for your physical heart and your spiritual heart. It removes stress, opens your heart to love and be loved, makes you less angry and less depressed.

As a physician, I see many people who are trying to solve spiritual problems with medical solutions, but ultimately it can't be done. Doctors may be able to take away some of the symptoms of a spiritual or emotional problem, but the problem itself will remain until it is recognized and dealt with in the heart and mind.

Do you have chronic fears? A hostile attitude? Unexplained or uncontrolled sadness or depression? There are alternatives that may control your stress and depression. Accepting Bible principles may not resolve the problem completely, but Jesus is the only one who can truly take away the fear. His Word says, "The LORD is my light and my salvation; whom shall I fear? The LORD is the strength of my life; of whom shall I be afraid?" (Ps. 27:1, KJV). In Him there is no *ultimate* fear because only He guarantees your ticket to heaven.

Have you considered giving your heart to Christ? Every physical heart will eventually give way, but your spiritual heart will live forever. Physical solutions are temporary; spiritual solutions are eternal. If you died today, are you absolutely sure what would happen and where you would end up?

Why not give your spiritual heart to Christ and see your body and soul flourish with health? The Bible says that all have sinned and fallen short of the glory of God, but that in

Christ we can be born again and leave our old life behind. (See Romans 3:23.) When we put our lives in Jesus' hands, we become new creatures. Our spiritual hearts are transformed and made new.

Your spiritual heart is vastly more important than the beating pump inside your chest. Indeed, the physical heart is really a picture of the spiritual heart, giving life to our bodies, keeping us healthy and fit. Of all the advice I have for you, this is the most important by far: Let your heart find rest in God and accept His gift of salvation through Jesus Christ. Your spiritual and physical hearts will never be the same.

In this book we have discussed many ways to protect the heart: eating healthy, exercising, chelation therapy, nurturing our emotional and spiritual hearts and avoiding bad habits like smoking, excessive drinking and overeating.

Nevertheless, a healthy heart is the result not just of doing the "dos" and avoiding the "don'ts," but building a lifestyle that is enjoyable to you and is heart-healthy all at once. You now have the power and the keys to change your life, to lengthen and enrich it. And you have the opportunity to give your spiritual heart to Christ so that when your physical heart finally gives out you will have a permanent home in heaven.

I pray that you will be blessed for years to come with a healthy physical heart, a healthy spiritual heart and a life rich with the best God has to offer you.

Notes

CHAPTER 1
WHAT IS HEART DISEASE?

1. Source obtained from the Internet: "The History of Heart Disease," The Franklin Institute Online, www.fi.edu/biosci/history/history.html.
2. National Center for Health Statistics, "Leading Causes of Death 1900–1978" (Hyattsville, MD: Public Health Service).
3. Ibid.
4. See note 1.
5. Ronald M. Lauer et al., "National Cholesterol Education Program," *Pediatrics* (March 1992): 530.
6. Source obtained from the Internet: "American Heart Disease," The Franklin Institute Online, www.fi.edu/biosci/healthy/stats.html.
7. Source obtained from the Internet: Thomas Jefferson University Hospital, www.jeffersonhospital.org/hearts/show.asp?durki=4017.
8. Source obtained from the Internet: American Heart Association, www.americanheart.org.
9. See note 7.
10. See note 8.
11. See note 7.
12. Source obtained from the Internet: The Franklin Institute Online, www.fi.edu.
13. See note 7.
14. Ibid.
15. Barry L. Zaret, Marvin, Moser, Lawrence S. Cohen, eds., *Yale University School of Medicine Heart Book* (New York: William Morrow and Company, Inc., n.d.), 237.
16. Source obtained from the Internet: Judith Larosa, "Testimony of the American Heart Association," American Heart Association (July 22, 1997): www.americanheart.org/support/advocacy/research/womhealth.html.
17. Zaret et al., *Yale University School of Medicine Heart Book*, 237.
18. See note 16.
19. Source obtained from the Internet: The Franklin Institute Online, www.fi.edu.
20. *World Book Encyclopedia*, software version 1.0, 1998, s.v. "heart."
21. Ibid.
22. Source obtained from the Internet: Charles A. Andersen, M.D., "Understanding Your Atherosclerosis and Living With It," *Iowa Health Book: Internal Medicine*, www.vh.org/patients/ihb/intmed/cardio/athero/atherosclerosis.html.

23. Zaret et al., *Yale University School of Medicine Heart Book*, 136.
24. Ibid.
25. Ibid., 143.
26. Ibid.
27. Ibid.
28. See note 6.
29. See note 22.
30. Zaret et al., *Yale University School of Medicine Heart Book*, 239
31. Ibid., 240.
32. Ibid., 245.
33. Ibid., 241.
34. Ibid.
35. Ibid.
36. Source obtained from the Internet: Suzanne Rostler, "Clerical jobs linked to heart disease risk," Reuters Ltd., Center for Cardiovascular Education, Inc., www.heartinfo.org.
37. Zaret et al., *Yale University School of Medicine Heart Book*, 242.
38. Ibid., 243.
39. Eva Prescott et al., "Smoking and risk of myocardial infarction in women and men: longitudinal population study," *British Medical Journal* 316, 7137 (April 4, 1998); Press release, *British Medical Journal* (April 2, 1998); source obtained from the Internet: Reuters Health Information Services, Inc., Reuters Ltd., Center for Cardiovascular Education, Inc. (April 4, 1998): www.heartinfo.org.

CHAPTER 2
TREATING HEART DISEASE

1. Source obtained from the Internet: The Franklin Institute Online, www.fi.edu.
2. Source obtained from the Internet: The Learning Kingdom, Inc., copyright 2000, http://features/learningKingdom.com/fact/archive/2000/03/08.html.
   Also, *The Hutchinson Family Encyclopedia* (Helicon Publishing Ltd., 2000).
3. Source obtained from the Internet: Thomas Jefferson University Hospital, www.jeffersonhospital.org/hearts/show.asp?durki=4017.
4. Source obtained from the Internet: "Deadliest Creature: Sea Wasp," www.extremescience.com/deadliestcreature.htm.
5. *World Book Encyclopedia,* software version 1.0, 1998, s.v. "heart."
6. Zaret et al., *Yale University School of Medicine Heart Book*, 134.
7. Source obtained from the Internet: Charles A. Andersen, M.D., "Understanding Your Atherosclerosis and Living With It," *Iowa Health Book: Internal Medicine*, www.vh.org/patients/ihb/intmed/cardio/athero/atherosclerosis.html.
8. Source obtained from the Internet: The Franklin Institute Online,

www.fi.edu.

9. Ibid.

10. Ibid. Also see note 3.

11. See note 3.

12. Source obtained from the Internet: The Angioplasty/PTCA Home Page, www.ptca.org/history.html.

13. AP, "Angioplasty beats clot-busters—sometimes," *Sacramento Bee* (December 27, 2000): A9.

14. Source obtained from the Internet: The Franklin Institute Online, www.fi.edu.

15. Source obtained from the Internet: "Building a Better Heart," The Franklin Institute Online, www.fi.edu/biosci/ healthy/fake.html.

16. Raja Mishra, "A Heartbeat Away," *San Diego Tribune* (February 14, 2001): F5.

CHAPTER 3
AT THE MERCY OF TECHNOLOGY

1. Thomas J. Moore, *Heart Failure: A Critical Inquiry Into American Medicine and the Revolution in Heart Care* (New York: Random House, n.d.), 106.

2. Ibid., 153; also, source obtained from the Internet: Louise Williams, "Framingham Heart Study Celebrates 50 Years," NIH Record (November 17, 1998): www.nih.gov/news/NIH-Record/11_17_98/story06.htm.

3. Moore, *Heart Failure,* 153.

4. L. Kristin Newby, M.D., et al., "The Chest Pain Unit—Ready for Prime Time?", *New England Journal of Medicine* (December 24, 1998): 1930.

5. Lisa M. Schwartz et al., "Misunderstanding about the Effects of Race and Sex on Physicians' Referrals for Cardiac Catheterization," *New England Journal of Medicine* (July 22, 1999): 281.

6. Mridu Gulati, M.D. et al., "Impatient Inpatient Care," *New England Journal of Medicine* (January 6, 2000): 39–40.

7. Source obtained from the Internet: William E. Boden et al., "Outcomes in Patients with Acute Non-Q-Wave Myocardial Infarction Randomly Assigned to an Invasive as Compared with a Conservative Management Strategy," *New England Journal of Medicine* (June 18, 1998): www.nejm.org/content/1998/0338/0025/1785.asp.

8. Heiner C. Bucher et al., "Percutaneous transluminal coronary angioplasty versus medical treatment for non-acute coronary heart disease: meta-analysis of randomized controlled trials," *British Medical Journal.*

9. Moore, *Heart Failure,* 270–271.

10. Source obtained from the Internet: L. S. Piegas et al., "The Organization to Assess Strategies for Ischemic Syndromes (OASIS)

registry in patients with unstable angina," Instituto Dante
Pazzanese de Cardiologia, Sao Paulo, SP, Brazil. *Am J Cardiol* 84
(5A) (September 2, 1999): 7M–12M;
www.ncbi.nlm.nih.gov/htbin-post/Entrez/query/
?uid=10505537&form=6&db=m&Dopt=b.

11. Source obtained from the Internet: "Use and Overuse of
     Angiography and Revascularization for Acute Coronary
     Syndromes," *New England Journal of Medicine* (June 18, 1998):
     www.nejm.org/content/1998/0338/0025/1838.asp.

12. Ibid.

13. Ibid.

14. Howard H. Wayne, *Living Longer With Heart Disease: The
     Noninvasive Approach That Will Save Your Life* (Los Angeles:
     Health Information Press, 1998). Also,
     www.heartprotect.com/mortality-stats.shtml.

15. Ibid.

16. Source obtained from the Internet: P. Peduzzi, A. Kamina and K.
     Detre, "Twenty-two-year follow-up in the VA Cooperative Study of
     Coronary Artery Bypass Surgery for Stable Angina," *Am J Cardiol*
     81 (12) (June 15, 1998): 1393–1399; www.ncbi.nlm.nih.gov/htbin-
     post/Entrez/ query/?uid=9645886&form=6&db=m&Dopt=b.

17. James Gerstenzang, "Pains Prompt Urgent Heart Care for
     Cheney," *Los Angeles Times* (March 6, 2001): A1.

18. "Loss of brainpower after bypass may last," *USA Today* (February
     8, 2001): 10D.

19. Source obtained from the Internet: Alice K. Jacobs., M.D.,
     "Coronary Stents–Have They Fulfilled Their Promise?", *New
     England Journal of Medicine* (December 23, 1999):
     www.nejm.org/content/1999/0341/0026/2005.asp.

20. Ibid.

21. Source obtained from the Internet: Howard H. Wayne, M.D.,
     "Angiograms: Point of View–a Life or Death Matter," www.heart-
     protect.com/angiograms.shtml.

22. Ibid.

23. Barry Sears, Ph.D., *The Zone* (New York: HarperCollins, 1995),
     135.

24. Ibid.

25. Source obtained from the Internet: The Doctors' Guide,
     www.docguide.com.

26. Peggy C. W. van den Hoogen et al., "The Relation Between Blood
     Pressure and Mortality Due to Coronary Heart Disease Among
     Men in Different Parts of the World," *New England Journal of
     Medicine* 342, no. 1 (January 6, 2000), 7.

CHAPTER 4

THE STUNNING TRUTH ABOUT CHOLESTEROL

1. Source obtained from the Internet: Reuters Ltd., copyright ©
    1998, www.heartinfo.org/reuters2000/t021622f.htm.

2. Michael R. Eades, *Protein Power* (New York: Bantam, 1997), 362.

3. Ibid., 362–364.
4. Ibid., 392.
5. Ibid., 362–364.
6. Source obtained from the Internet: Uffe Ravnskov, M.D., "The Cholesterol Myths," home.swipnet.se/~w-25775/.
7. Source obtained from the Internet: "Locating Gene That Explains Cholesterol Absorption," University of Texas Southwestern Medical Center (September 1, 1998): www.newswise.com/articles/1998/9/ABSORB.SWM.html.
8. Moore, *Heart Failure*, 72.
9. Ibid., 71.
10. Ibid., 72.
11. Source obtained from the Internet: Uffe Ravnskov, M.D., "The Cholesterol Myths," home.swipnet.se/~w-25775/.
12. Ibid.
13. Ibid.
14. Ibid.
15. Artemis P. Simopoulos, M.D., and Jo Robinson, *The Omega Diet* (formerly published as *The Omega Plan*) (New York: HarperCollins, 1998), 50.
16. Sears, *The Zone*, 142.
17. See note 11.
18. Moore, *Heart Failure*, 95.
19. Ibid., 94.

CHAPTER 5
ARE YOU EATING HEART SMART?

1. Eades, *Protein Power*.
2. S. Bengmark, "Ecoimmunonutrition: A Challenge for the Third Millennium," *Nutrition* 14, no. 7–8 (1998): 563–572.
3. Rex Russell, M.D., *What the Bible Says About Healthy Living* (Ventura, CA: Regal Books, 1997).
4. U.S. Department of Health and Human Services, *The Surgeon General's Report on Nutrition and Health* (New York: Warner Books, 1989), 2.
5. Ibid., 2, 6.
6. Ibid., 19.
7. M. W. Gillman et al., "Protective effect of fruits and vegetables on development of stroke in men," *JAMA* 273 (1995): 1113–1117.
8. Peggy C. W. van den Hoogen et al., "The Relation Between Blood Pressure and Mortality Due to Coronary Heart Disease Among Men in Different Parts of the World," *New England Journal of Medicine* 342, no. 1 (January 6, 2000), 7.
9. Dean Ornish, M.D., "Low-Fat Diets," *New England Journal of Medicine* 338, no. 2 (January 8, 1998): 127.
10. C. L. Vecchia, A. Decareli and R. Pagano, "Vegetable consumption and risk of chronic disease," *Epidemiology* 9 (1998): 208–210.

11. F. Sacks et al., "A dietary approach to prevent hypertension: a review of the dietary approaches to stop hypertension (DASH) study," *Clinical Cardiology* 22, Supplement III (1999): III-6–III-10.

12. B. V. Howard and D. Kritchevsky, "Phytochemicals and cardiovascular disease: a statement for health care professionals from the American Heart Association," *Circulation* 95 (1997): 2591–2593.

13. C. V. DeWhalley et al., "Flavonoids inhibit the oxidative modification of low-density lipoproteins by macrophages," *Biochemistry and Pharmacology* 39 (1990): 1743–1750.

14. M. G. L. Hertog et al., "Dietary antioxidant flavonoids and risk of coronary heart disease: the Zutphen Elderly Study," *The Lancet* 342 (1993): 1077–1011.

15. L. Yochum et al., "Dietary flavonoid intake and risk of cardiovascular disease in postmenopausal women," *American Journal of Epidemiology* 149 (1999): 943–949.

16. R. A. Nagourney, "Garlic: Medicinal food or nutritious medicine?", *Journal of Medicinal Food* 1, no. 1 (1998): 13–28.

17. W. J. Graig, "Phytochemicals: Guardians of Our Health," *Journal of the American Dietetic Association* 97, Supplement 2 (1997): S199–S204.

18. Ibid.

19. F. Visoli et al., "Low-density lipoprotein oxidation is inhibited in vitro by olive oil constituents," *Atherosclerosis* 117 (1995): 25–32. F. Visoli, G. Bellomo and C. Galli, "Free-radical-scavenging properties of olive oil polyphenols," *Biochem. Biophys. Res. Comm.* 247 (1998): 60–64.

20. "Olive oil may reduce need for blood pressure drugs," *Archives of Internal Medicine* 160 (2000): 837–842; Center for Cardiovascular Education, Inc., Reuters Ltd., www.heartinfo.org.

21. G. E. Fraser et al., "A possible protective effect of nut consumption on risk of coronary heart disease," *Archives of Internal Medicine* 152 (1992): 1416–1424. L. Brown, "Nut consumption and risk of recurrent coronary heart disease (abstract)," *FASEB Journal* 13, no. 4–5 (1999): A538.

22. G. E. Fraser, K. D. Lindsted and W. L. Beeson, "Effect of risk factor values on lifetime risk of an age at first coronary event," *American Journal of Epidemiology* 142 (1995): 746–758.

23. D. Steinberg and A. Lewis, "Oxidative modification of LDL and atherogenesis," *Circulation* 95 (1997): 1062–1071.

24. J. G. Keevil, "Grape juice, but not orange juice or grapefruit juice, inhibit human platelet aggregation," *Journal of Nutrition* 130 (2000): 53–56.

25. R. Sauter, J. D. Folts and J. E. Freedman, "Purple grape juice inhibits platelet function and increases platelet-derived nitric oxide release," *Circulation* 98 (1998): 581–585.

26. W. B. Kannel and R. C. Ellison, "Alcohol and coronary heart disease: the evidence for a protective effect," *Clin. Chim. Acta* 246 (1996): 59–76.

27. D. R. Lowry et al., "Alcohol consumption and incidence of hypertension: The John Hopkins Precursors Study," *Circulation* 92, no. 8 (1995): 619.

28. G. J. Soleas, E. P. Diamandis and D. M. Goldberg, "Wine as a biological fluid: History, production, and role in disease prevention," *Journal of Clinical Laboratory Analysis* 11 (1997): 287–313.

29. S. V. Nigdikar et al., "Consumption of red wine polyphenols reduces the susceptibility of low-density lipoproteins to oxidation in vivo," *American Journal of Clinical Nutrition* 68 (1998): 258–265.

30. S. Renaud and M.de Lorgeril, "Wine, alcohol, platelets and the French paradox for coronary heart disease," *The Lancet* 339 (1992): 1523–1526.

31. J. M. Geleijnse et al., "Tea flavonoids may protect against atheroesclerosis: The Rotterdam Study," *Arch. Inter. Med.* 159 (1999): 2170–2174.

32. A. A. Hakim et al., "Coffee consumption in hypertensive men in older middle-age and the risk of stroke: The Honolulu Heart Program," *Journal of Clinical Epidemiology* 51, no. 6 (1998): 487–494.

33. M. Woodward and H. Tunstall-Pedoe, "Coffee and tea consumption in the Scottish Heart Health Study follow-up: conflicting relations with coronary risk factors, coronary disease, and all cause mortality," *Journal of Epidemiology Community Health* 53 (1999): 481–487.

34. C. Sanbongi, N. Suzuki and T. Sakane, "Polyphenols in chocolate, which have antioxidant activity, modulate immune functions in humans in vitro," *Cellular Immunology* 177 (1997): 129–136.

35. A. L. Waterhouse, J. R. Shirley and J. L. Donovan, "Antioxidants in chocolate," *The Lancet* 348 (1996): 384.

36. P. N. Appleby et al., "The Oxford Vegetarian Study: an overview," *American Journal of Clinical Nutrition* 70, Supplement (1999): 525S–531S.

37. E. J. Schaefer and M. E. Brosseau, "Diet, lipoproteins, and coronary heart disease," *Endocrinology and Metabolism Clinics of North America* 27, no. 3 (1998): 711–732.

38. G. M. Wardlaw and T. J. Snook, "Effect of diets high in butter, corn oil, or high-oleic acid sunflower oil or serum lipids and apolipoproteins in men," *American Journal of Clinical Nutrition* 51 (1990): 815–822. P. Mata, J. A. Garrido and J. M. Ordovas, "Effect of dietary monounsaturated fatty acids on plasma lipoproteins and apolipoproteins in women," *American Journal of Clinical Nutrition* 56 (1992): 77–83.

39. Russell, *What the Bible Says About Healthy Living*, 135.
40. E. B. Rimm et al., "Vegetable, fruit, and cereal intake and risk of coronary heart disease among men," *JAMA* 275 (1996): 447–451.
41. G. E. Fraser et al., "A possible protective effect of nut consumption on risk of coronary heart disease: the Adventist Health Study," *Archives in Internal Medicine* 152 (1992): 1416–1424.
42. D. R. Jacobs, Jr. et al., "Whole-grain intake may reduce the risk of ischemic heart disease death in postmenopausal women: the Iowa Women's Health Study," *American Journal of Clinical Nutrition* 68 (1998): 248–257.
43. S. Liu et al., "Whole-grain consumption and risk of coronary heart disease: results from the Nurses' Health Study," *American Journal of Clinical Nutrition* 70 (1999): 412–419.
44. S. Liu et al., "Methodological considerations in applying metabolic data to an epidemiologic study using a semi-quantitative food frequency questionnaire," *European Journal of Clinical Nutrition* 52 (1998): S87.
45. W. E. Connor, "Importance of n-3 fatty acids in health and disease," *American Journal of Clinical Nutrition* 71, Supplement (2000): 171S–175S.
46. D. S. Siscovick et al., "Dietary intake of long-chain n-3 polyunsaturated fatty acids and the risk of primary cardiac arrest," *American Journal of Clinical Nutrition* 71, Supplement (2000): 208S–212S. H. O. Bang, J. Dyerberg and H. M. Sinclair, "The composition of the Eskimo food in north western Greenland," *American Journal of Clinical Nutrition* 33 (1980): 2657–2661.
47. D. S. Siscovick et al., "Dietary intake of long-chain n-3 polyunsaturated fatty acids and the risk of primary cardiac arrest," *American Journal of Clinical Nutrition* 71, Supplement (2000): 208S–212S.
48. F. N. Hepburn, J. Exler and J. L. Weilharach, "Provisional tables on the content of omega-3 fatty acids and other fat components of selected foods," *Journal of the American Diet Association* 86 (1986): 788–793. S. L. Connor and W. E. Connor, "Are fish oils beneficial in the prevention and treatment of coronary artery disease?", *American Journal of Clinical Nutrition* 66, Supplement (1997): 1020S–1031S.
49. P. M. Kris-Etherton et al., "Polyunsaturated fatty acids in the food chain in the United States," *American Journal of Clinical Nutrition* 71, Supplement (2000): 179S–188S.
50. J. X. Kang and A. Leaf, "Prevention of fatal arrhythmias by polyunsaturated fatty acids," *American Journal of Clinical Nutrition* 71, Supplement (2000): 202S–207S.
51. See note 47.
52. M. L. Burr et al., "Effects of changes in fat, fish, and fiber intakes on death and myocardial reinfarction: Diet and Reinfarction Trial

(DART)," *The Lancet* 2 (1989): 756–761.

53. M. DeLorgeril et al., "Mediterranean alpha-linolenic acid-rich diet secondary prevention of coronary heart disease," *The Lancet* 343 (1994): 1454–1459.
54. C. M. Albert et al., "Fish consumption and risk of sudden cardiac death," *JAMA* 279 (1998): 23–27.
55. Simopoulos, *The Omega Diet*, 52.
56. H. Shimokawa and P. M. Vanhoutte, "Dietary omega-3 fatty acids and endothelium-dependent relaxations in porcine coronary arteries," *American Journal of Physiology* 256 (1989): H968–H973.
57. Simopoulos, *The Omega Diet*, 52–53, 102.
58. Ibid., 95.
59. See note 45 and note 47.

CHAPTER 6
CHOOSING A HEART-SMART EATING LIFESTYLE

1. Russell, *What the Bible Says About Healthy Living*, 177.
2. Ibid.
3. D. L. Ely, "Overview of dietary sodium effects on and interactions with cardiovascular and neuroendocrine functions," *American Journal of Clinical Nutrition* 65, Supplement (1997): 594S-605S.
4. Ibid.
5. G. S. Chrysant, S. Bakir and S. Oparil, "Dietary salt reduction in hypertension—what is the evidence and why is it still controversial?", *Progress in Cardiovascular Diseases* 42, no.1 (1999): 23-38. J. G. Fodor et al., "Recommendations on dietary salt," *Canadian Medical Association Journal* 160, Supplement 9 (1999): S29–S34.
6. See note 3 and note 5.
7. J. G. Fodor et al., "Recommendations on dietary salt," *Canadian Medical Association Journal* 160, Supplement 9 (1999): S29–S34.
8. See note 5.
9. See note 7.
10. Alberto Ascherio, M.D. et al., "Trans Fatty Acids and Coronary Heart Disease," *New England Journal of Medicine* (June 24, 1999), 1997.
11. Source obtained from the Internet: People for the Ethical Treatment of Animals (PETA), www.meatstinks.com.
12. Source obtained from the Internet: Julie Brussell, "Traditional Foods, Unconventional Wisdom," *Conscious Choice* (September 2000): www.consciouschoice.com/issues/cc1309/traditional-foods1309.html.
13. Source obtained from the Internet: Sally Fallon, "Nasty, brutish and short," The Weston A. Price Foundation, www.weston-aprice.org/nasty_brutish_short.htm.
14. Source obtained from the Internet: Staffan Lindeberg, "On the Benefits of Ancient Diets," www.panix.com/~paleodiet/lindeberg/.

15. Source obtained from the Internet: Riccardo Baschetti, "Diabetes in aboriginal populations," *Canadian Medical Association Journal* 162 (2000): 969; www.cma.ca/cmaj/vol-162/issue-7/0969a.htm.

16. Source obtained from the Internet: Press release, "Traditional Chinese Diet Helps Ward Off Heart Disease," www.cuhk.edu.hk/ipro/991110e.htm.

17. Source obtained from the Internet: Sarah Yang, "Mediterranean diet still healthy when authentic, not Americanized," CNN.com republished article by WebMD, www2.cnn.com/2000/FOOD/news/05/01/mediterranean.eating.wmd/index.html.

18. A. Trichopoulou and P. Lagiou, "Healthy traditional Mediterranean diet: An expression of culture, history and lifestyle," *Nutrition Reviews* 55, no.11 (1997): 383-389.

19. Ibid.

20. S. Renaud, et al., "Cretan Mediterranean diet for prevention of coronary heart disease," *American Journal of Clinical Nutrition* 61, Supplement 6 (1995): 1360S-1637S.

CHAPTER 7
BOOST HEART POWER WITH
SUPPLEMENTS, ASPIRIN AND HORMONES

1. Source obtained from the Internet: M. Rene Malinow et al., "Homocysteine, Diet, and Cardiovascular Diseases," American Heart Association, www.americanheart.org/Scientific/statements/1999/019901.html.

2. Ibid.

3. P. L. Canner et al., "Fifteen year mortality in coronary drug project patients: Long term benefit with niacin," *Journal of the American College of Cardiology* 8 (1986): 1245–1255. M. H. Luria, "Effect of low-dose niacin on high-density lipoprotein cholesterol and total cholesterol/high-density lipoprotein cholesterol ratio," *Archives of Internal Medicine* 148 (1998): 2493–2495.

4. E. B. Rimm et al., "Folate and vitamin B6 from diet and supplements in relation to risk of coronary heart disease among women," *JAMA* 279, no.5 (1998): 359–364.

5. M. J. Stampfer et al., "A prospective study of plasma homocysteine and risk of myocardial infarction in US physicians," *JAMA* 268, no.7 (1992): 877–881.

6. See note 4.

7. B. Frei, L. England and B. N. Ames, "Ascorbate is an outstanding antioxidant in human blood plasma," Proceedings of the *National Academy of Science USA* 86, (1989): 6377–6381. A. K. Bordia, "The effect of vitamin C on blood lipids, fibrinolytic activity and platelet adhesiveness in patients with coronary artery disease," *Atheroesclerosis* 35, (1980): 181–187.

8. Thomas H. Maugh II, "High Vitamin C Levels in Blood Are Found

Beneficial," *Los Angeles Times* (March 5, 2001): S3.

9. Ibid.

10. S. P. Azen, et al., "Effect of supplementary antioxidant vitamin intake on carotid arterial wall intima-media thickness in a controlled clinical trial of cholesterol lowering," *Circulation* 94 (1996): 2369–2372.

11. E. B. Rimm et al., "Vitamin E consumption and the risk of coronary heart disease onset in men," *New England Journal of Medicine* 328 (1993): 1450–1456.

12. A possible mechanism is the following: Low serum calcium would increase the constriction of arterioles (reducing their diameter), which in turn increases arterial resistance to blood flow. As a result, blood pressure is increased.

13. P. Hamet, "The evaluation of the scientific evidence for a relationship between calcium and hypertension," *Journal of Nutrition* 125, Supplement 2 (1995): 311S–400S.

14. L. J. Appel et al., "A clinical trial of the effects of dietary patterns on blood pressure," *New England Journal of Medicine* 336 (1997): 1117–1124.

15. M. F. McCarty, "Hypothesis: sensitization of insulin-dependent hypothalamic glucoreceptors may account for the fat-reducing effects of chromium picolinate," *Journal of Optimal Nutrition* 2, no. 1 (1993): 36–53.

16. Ibid.

17. M. Simonoff, Y. Llabador, C. Hamon et al., "Low plasma chromium in patients with coronary artery and heart disease," *Biol Trace Elen Res* 6 (1984): 431–439.

18. M. Shechter et al., "Beneficial effects of magnesium sulfate in acute myocardial infarction," *American Journal of Cardiology* 66 (1990): 271–274.

19. Ibid.

20. M. S. Neff et al., "Magnesium sulfate in digitalis toxicity," *American Journal of Cardiology* 29 (1972): 377–382.

21. P. K. Whelton et al., "Effects of oral potassium on blood pressure: Meta-analysis of randomized controlled clinical trials," *JAMA* 277, no. 20 (1997): 1624–1632.

22. A. Kalen, E. L. Appelkvist and G. Dallner, "Age-related changes in the lipid compositions of rat and human tissues," *Lipids* 24 (1989): 579–581.

23. A. Kontush et al., "Plasma ubiquinol-10 is decreased in patients with hyperlipidaemia," *Atherosclerosis* 129 (1997): 119–126. K. Folkers, G. P. Littarru and L. Ho, "Evidence for a deficiency of coenzyme Q10 in human heart disease," *Int. J. Vitamin. Nutr. Res.* 40 (1970): 380–390.

24. S. T. Sinatra, "Coenzyme Q10: A vital therapeutic nutrient for the heart with special application in congestive heart failure,"

Connecticut Medicine 61, no. 11 (1997): 707–711.

25. R. B. Singh et al., "Randomized, double-blind placebo-controlled trial of coenzyme Q10 in patients with acute myocardial infarction," *Cardiovascular Drugs and Therapy* 12 (1998): 347–353.

26. R. B. Singh and M. A. Niaz, "Serum concentration of lipoprotein(a) decreases on treatment with hydrosoluble coenzyme Q10 in patients with coronary artery disease: discovery of a new role," *International Journal of Cardiology* 68 (1999): 23–29.

27. A. Z. Reznick et al., "Antiradical effects in L-propionyl carnitine protection of the heart against ischemia-reperfusion injury: the possible role of iron chelation," *Arch Biochem. Biophys.* 296 (1992): 394–401.R. B. Singh et al., "A randomized, double-blind, placebo-controlled trial of L-carnitine in suspected acute myocardial infarction," *Postgrad. Med. Journal* 72 (1996): 45–60.

28. J. Arenas J et al., "Carnitine in muscle, serum and urine of non-professional athletes: Effects of physical exercise, training, and L-carnitine administration," *Muscle and Nerve* 14 (1991): 598–604.

29. B. Wittels and J. F. Spann, "Defective lipid metabolism in the failing heart," *Journal of Clinical Investigation* 47 (1968): 1787–1794.

30. A. Z. Reznick et al., "Antiradical effects in L-propionyl carnitine protection of the heart against ischemia-reperfusion injury: the possible role of iron chelation," *Arch Biochem. Biophys.* 296 (1992): 394–401.

31. R. B. Singh et al., "A randomized, double-blind, placebo-controlled trial of L-carnitine in suspected acute myocardial infarction," *Postgrad. Med. Journal* 72 (1996): 45–60.

32. See note 30.

33. T. Kamikawa et al., "Effects of L-carnitine on exercise tolerance in patients with stable angina pectoris," *Japanese Heart Journal* 25 (1984): 587–597.

34. V. Diglesi et al., "L-carnitine adjuvant therapy in essential hypertension," *Clin. Ther.* 5 (1994): 391–395.

35. I. Anand et al., "Acute and chronic effects of propionyl-L-carnitine on the hemodynamics, exercise capacity, and hormones in patients with congestive heart failure," *Cardiovascular Drugs and Therapy* 12 (1998): 291–299. A. Kobayashi, Y. Masumura and N. Yamazaki, "L-carnitine treatment for congestive heart failure: Experimental and clinical study," *Japanese Circulation Journal* 56 (1992): 86–94.

36. M. Maebashi et al., "Lipid-lowering effect of carnitine in patients with type-IV Hyperlipoproteinaemia," *Lancet* 2 (1978): 805–807.

37. S. Iliceto et al., "Effect of L-carnitine administration on left ventricular remodeling after acute anterior myocardial infarction: The L-carnitine ecocardiografia digitalizzata infarto miocardio (CEDIM) trial," *Journal of the American College of Cardiology* 26, no. 2 (1995): 380–387. R. Sethi et al., "Beneficial effects of propionyl L-carnitine on sarcolemnal changes in congestive heart failure due to

myocardial infarction," *Cardiovascular Research* 42 (1999): 607–615.

38. G. Brevetti et al., "Propionyl-L-carnitine in intermittent claudication: Double-blind, placebo-controlled, dose titration, multicenter study," *Journal of the American College of Cardiology* 26, no.6 (1995): 1411–1416.

39. See notes 33, 35 and 38.

40. N. Awata et al., "Acute haemodyonamic effect of taurine on hearts in vivo with normal and depressed myocardial function," *Cardiovascular Research* 21 (1987): 241–247.

41. A. Sawamura et al. "Protection by oral pretreatment with taurine against the negative inotropic effects of low calcium medium on isolated perfused chick heart," *Cardiovascular Research* 17 (1983): 620. See note 40.

42. J. Azuma et al., "Therapeutic effect of taurine in congestive heart failure: a double-blind crossover trial," *Clin. Cardiol* 8, no.5 (1985): 276–282. J. Azuma, "Long-term effect of taurine in congestive heart failure: Preliminary report," in R. Huxtable and D. V. Michalk, ed., *Taurine in Health and Disease* (New York: Plenum Press, 1994), 425–433.

43. T. Nakamura et al., "The protective effect of taurine on the biomembrane against damage produced by oxygen radicals," *Biol. Pharm. Bull.* 16 (1993): 970–972.

44. See note 41 and note 40.

45. M. J. Meldrum et al., "The effect of taurine on blood pressure, and urinary sodium, potassium and calcium excretion," in Huxtable, *Taurine in Health and Disease*, 207–215.

46. See note 41 and note 40.

47. H. Yokogoshi et al., "Dietary taurine enhances cholesterol degradation and reduces serum and liver cholesterol concentrations in rats fed a high-cholesterol diet," *Journal of Nutrition* 129 (1999): 1705–1712.

48. Ibid.

49. J. Azuma and A. Sawamura, "Usefulness of taurine in chronic congestive heart failure and its prospective application," *Japanese Circulation Journal* 56 (1992): 95–99. J. Azuma, "Long-term effect of taurine in congestive heart failure: Preliminary report," in Huxtable, *Taurine in Health and Disease*, 425–433.

50. R. Shanthi et al., "Effect of tincture of Crataegus on the LDL-Receptor activity of hepatic plasma membrane of rats fed an atherogenic diet," *Atheroesclerosis* 123 (1996): 235–241. S. Pöpping et al., "Effect of a hawthorn extract on contraction and energy turnover of isolated rat cardiomyocytes," *Arzneimittel-Forschung/Drug Research* 45 (II), no. 11 (1995): 1157–1160.

51. M. Tauchert, A. Gildor and J. Lipinski, "High-dose Crataegus extract WS 1442 treatment of NYHA stage II heart failure," *Herz*

24, no.6 (1999): 465–474.

52. M. Sato et al., "Cardioprotective effects of grape seed proantho-cyanidin against ischemic reperfusion injury," *Journal of Molecular and Cellular Cardiology* 31 (1999): 1289–1297.

53. K. Welt, G. Fitzl and L. Schaffranietz, "Myocardium–protective effects of ginkgo biloba extract (EGb 761) in old rats against acute isobaric hypoxia. An electron microscopic morphometric study. II Protection of microvascular endothelium," *Exp. Toxic. Pathol.* 48 (1996): 81–86.

54. M. Steiner et al., "A double-blind crossover study in moderately hypercholesterolemic men that compared the effect of aged garlic extract and placebo administration on blood lipids," *American Journal of Clinical Nutrition* 64 (1996): 866–870. B. Reitz et al., "Cardioprotective action of wild garlic (allium ursinum) in schemia and reperfusion," *Mol. Cell Biochem.* 119 (1993): 143–150.

55. Sears, *The Zone*, 114.

56. Zaret et al., *Yale University School of Medicine Heart Book*, 281, 141.

57. Ibid., 243.

58. Ibid., 145.

59. Burton Goldberg, *Alternative Medicine. The Definitive Guide* (Tiburon, CA: Future Medicine Publishing, Inc., 1999), 718.

Chapter 8
Weighing In for Heart Health

1. Source obtained from the Internet: Matthew Waite, "A diner's huge appetite tests limits and tempers at a buffet restaurant," *St. Petersburg Times* (April 17, 2001): www.sptimes.com:80/News/041701/TampaBay/All_you_can_eatand_ea.shtml.

2. Erin Bried, *Self* (December 2000): 158–161.

3. Source obtained from the Internet: NIH Publication No. 96-4158 (July 1996, updated June 2000), the Weight-Control Information Network (WIN), a service of the National Institute of Diabetes and Digestive and Kidney Diseases (NIDDK), part of the National Institutes of Health under the U. S. Department of Health and Human Services, www.niddk.nih.gov/health/nutrit/pubs/statobes.htm# other.

4. Source obtained from the Internet: "Obesity Continues Climb in 1999 Among American Adults," (March 23, 2001): www.cdc.gov/nccdphp/dnpa/pr-obesity.htm.

5. Source obtained from the Internet: Suzanne Rostler, "Americans in denial about weight and risks of obesity," Reuters Ltd., Center for Cardiovascular Education, Inc., www.heartinfo.org.

6. *The Surgeon General's Report on Nutrition and Health*, 11.

7. Bried, *Self* (December 2000): 160–161.

8. Jerome Kassirer, "Losing Weight—an Ill-fated New Year's Resolution," *New England Journal of Medicine* (January 1, 1998): 53.
9. J. E. Manson et al., "Body weight and mortality among women," *New England Journal of Medicine* 333 (1995): 677–685. E. B. Rimm et al., "Body size and fat distribution as predictors of coronary heart disease among middle-aged and older U.S. men," *Am. J. Epidemiol.* 141 (1995): 1117–1127.
10. Source obtained from the Internet: www.heartinfo.org/ news97/obeshrt101597.htm.
11. Source obtained from the Internet: Adapted from Obesity Education Initiative: Clinical Guidelines on the Identification, Evaluation, and Treatment of Overweight and Obesity in Adults, National Institutes of Health, National Heart, Lung, and Blood Institute (June 1998): www.americanheart.org.
12. L. Lapidus et al., "Distribution of adipose tissue and risk of cardiovascular disease and death: a 12-year follow-up of participants in the population study of women in Gothenburg, Sweden," *BMJ* 289 (1984): 1257–1261. B. Larsson et al., "Abdominal adipose tissue distribution, obesity, and risk of cardiovascular disease and death: a 13-year follow-up of participants in the study of men born in 1913," *BMJ* 288 (1984): 1401–1404.
13. Source obtained from the Internet: Lynn Grieger, "Body Fat Distribution and Heart Disease Risk in Children and Adolescents," www.heartinfo.org/news99/ fatdist030399.htm.
14. Source obtained from the Internet: "Cholesterol and Children," WellnessWeb, www.wellweb.com/ smart/aahtchil.htm.
15. "National Cholesterol Education Program," *Pediatrics* (March 1992): 530.
16. The Bogalusa Heart Study, 2.
17. Richard P. Troiano, Ph.D. et al., "Overweight prevalence and Trends," *Arch Pediatr Adolesc Med* (October 1995): 1085, 1088.
18. See note 13.
19. Source obtained from the Internet: "Exercise, Lipids, and Obesity in Adolescents of Parents with Premature Coronary Disease," www.jhbmc.jhu.edu/cardiology/partnership/kids/ chdchildren/tsld034.htm.
20. Gerald S. Berenson, M.D. et al., "Association Between Multiple Cardiovascular Risk Factors and Atherosclerosis in Children and Young Adults," *New England Journal of Medicine* (June 4, 1998): 1655.
21. Source obtained from the Internet: "Cholesterol-lowering diets and effects on children," *Nutrition Today* (March 2000): www.findarticles.com/m0841/2_35/62083816/p1/ article.jhtml.

CHAPTER 9
EXERCISE—A FIT BODY FOR A TIRELESS HEART

1. Source obtained from the Internet: Thomas Jefferson University

Hospital, www.jeffersonhospital.org/hearts/
show.asp?durki=4017.

2. Ibid.

3. AP, "Study: Healthy living slashes heart risks," *Dallas Morning News* (November 9, 1999): 3A.

4. Ibid.

5. Janice C. Wright, "Gains in Life Expectancy from Medical Interventions—Standardizing Data on Outcomes," *New England Journal of Medicine* (August 6, 1998): 380–385.

6. Bried, *Self* (December 2000): 158.

7. Amy A. Hakim, et al., "Effects of Walking on Mortality Among Nonsmoking Retired Men," *New England Journal of Medicine* (January 8, 1998): 94–99.

8. Source obtained from the Internet: "Women put best foot forward to reduce heart disease, stroke risk," American Heart Association, www.americanheart.org/Whats_News_AHA_News_Releases/manson.htm.

9. Source obtained from the Internet: BBC, "Health Lifestyle Survey," news2.thls.bbc.co.uk/hi/english/health/newsid_258000/258580.stm.

10. Source obtained from the Internet: "Change in Coronary Risk and Coronary Risk Factor Levels in Couples Following Lifestyle Intervention," *Archives of Family Medicine* 6 (July/August 1997): 354–360; Reuters Ltd., July 21, 1997, Center for Cardiovascular Education, Inc., www.heartinfor.org.

CHAPTER 10

QUIT SMOKING FOR YOUR HEART'S SAKE

1. Source obtained from the Internet: Ira S. Ockene et al., "A Statement for Healthcare Professionals From the American Heart Association" (April 1997): www.americanheart.org.

2. Source obtained from the Internet: "Cigarette Smoking—Attributable Mortality and Years of Potential Life Lost—United States, 1990," 42, 33 (August 27, 1993): 645–649, www.cdc.gov/epo/mmwr/preview/mmwrhtml/00021441.htm.

3. Source obtained from the Internet: Denise Pinney, "Smoking series, part 1: Understanding the connection between smoking and heart disease," Reuters Ltd., Center for Cardiovascular Education, Inc., www.heartinfo.org.

4. "Understanding the connection between smoking and heart disease," "Cigarette smoking, cardiovascular disease, and stroke: A statement for healthcare professions from the American Heart Association," *Circulation: Journal of the American Heart Association* 96 (1997): 3243–3247.

5. Source obtained from the Internet: "Smoking said to promote clots," Reuters Ltd., Center for Cardiovascular Education, Inc., www.heartinfo.org.

6. Source obtained from the Internet: www.thehealthauthority.com/commons/ heartcare/ help_your_heart04.htm.

7. Source obtained from the Internet: "Every cigarette takes 11 minutes off man's life," Reuters Ltd., Center for Cardiovascular Education, Inc. www.heartinfo.org. Also, *British Medical Journal* 320 (2000): 53.

8. Source obtained from the Internet: "Passive smoke lowers vitamin C levels in children," Reuters, Ltd., Center for Cardiovascular Education, Inc., www.heartinfo.com. Also, *Pediatrics* 107 (2001): 540–542.

9. "Cigar smoking: an unsafe alternative to cigarettes," "Cigars to not have the same restrictions as cigarettes," *American Cancer Society News Today* (June 2000). Also, source obtained from the Internet: Reuters, Ltd., Center for Cardiovascular Education, Inc., www.heartinfo.com.

10. Ibid.

11. Ibid.

12. Source obtained from the Internet: Thomas Jefferson University Hospital, www.jeffersonhospital.org/hearts/ show.asp?durki=4017.

13. Source obtained from the Internet: www.smokeaway.org/whyquit.htm. Also, "Tobacco or Health: A Global Status Report," World Health Organization (1997), cited at www.americanheart.org.statistics/riskfactors.html#smoke.

14. Source obtained from the Internet: About.com, "Smoking and Your Smile," quitsmoking.miningco.com/health/ quitsmoking/library/weekly/aa052900a.htm.

CHAPTER 11
DON'T DEVELOP DIABETES OR HIGH BLOOD PRESSURE

1. Simopoulos, *The Omega Diet*, 51.

2. Zaret et al., *Yale University School of Medicine Heart Book,* 150–151.

3. Ibid., 157.

4. Ibid., 151.

5. Source obtained from the Internet: The Franklin Institute Online, www.fi.edu.

6. Source obtained from the Internet: Alicia Marie Belchak, "Exercise reduces heart disease among diabetics," *Annals of Internal Medicine* 134 (2001): 96–106; also, Reuters Ltd., Center for Cardiovascular Education, Inc., www.heartinfo.org.

7. Source obtained from the Internet: "Heart disease rates drop for all but diabetics," *The Journal of the American Medical Association* 281 (1999): 1291–1297; also, Reuters Ltd., Center for Cardiovascular Education, Inc., www.heartinfo.org.

8. Source obtained from the Internet: Emma Patten-Hitt, "Diabetic

arteries often re-close after surgery," *Circulation* 103 (2001): 1218–1224; also, Reuters Ltd., Center for Cardiovascular Education, Inc., www.heartinfo.org.

9. Source obtained from the Internet: Nancy Deutsch, "Link discovered between diabetes and heart disease," *The Journal of Clinical Investigation* 105 (2000): 1807–1818; also, Reuters Ltd., Center for Cardiovascular Education, Inc., www.heartinfo.org.

10. Source obtained from the Internet: Diabetes: A Growing Public Health Problem, www.cdc.gov/diabetes/ pubs/glance.htm#dcp.

11. Source obtained from the Internet: www.healthyideas.com/healing/cond_ail/diabetes2.html.

12. Ibid.

13. Source obtained from the Internet: American Diabetes Association, www.diabetes.org/ada/type2.asp.

14. Ibid.

15. See note 11.

Chapter 12
Don't Develop Gum Disease

1. F. Javier Nieto, "Infections and Atherosclerosis," *American Journal of Epidemiology* 148, no. 10.

2. Source from the Internet: Harvey Black, "The Connection Between Oral Health and Other Health," WebMD, onhealth.webmd.com/conditions/in-depth/item/ item%2C37240_1_1/asp.

3. Ibid.

4. Source obtained from the Internet: "Statement on the Link Between Gum Disease and Heart Disease," American Academy of Periodontology, www.perio.org/ consumer/webcardio.htm.

5. Source obtained from the Internet: Randolph Fillmore, "Gum Disease May Be a Threat to the Heart," WedMD, onhealth.webmd.com/conditions/in-depth/item/item.

6. Source obtained from the Internet: Judy Siegel-Itzkovich, "Gum disease can ruin far more than your smile," *Jerusalem Post* (June 25, 2000): 2; www.jpost.com/Editions/ 2000/05/21/Health/Health.6989.html.

7. Philippe P. Hujoel, Ph.D. et al., "Periodontal Disease and Coronary Heart Disease Risk," *JAMA* (September 20, 2000): 1409.

8. See note 5.

9. Ibid.

10. Ibid.

11. Tiejian Wu, M.D. et al., "Periodontal Disease and Risk of Cerebrovascular Disease," *Arch. Intern. Med.* 160 (October 9, 2000): 2753.

12. Eades, *Protein Power,* 397.

13. Jane Allen, "Link Between Infections and Heart Disease Bolstered," *Los Angeles Times* (March 5, 2001): S1.
14. See note 5. Also, "Another Reason to See the Dentist," WebMD (September 27, 1999): onhealth/webmd.com/conditions/briefs/item%2C50352.asp.
15. See note 5.
16. Source obtained from the Internet: Eurekalert, "Low dietary vitamin C can increase the risk for periodontal disease, especially in smokers," www.eurekalert.org/releases/aap-ldv081400.html.

CHAPTER 13
DETOXIFY YOUR ARTERIES WITH CHELATION

1. The result: He has enjoyed fifteen happy and healthy years beyond what other doctors said he would.
2. Dr. Morton Walker and Dr. Hitendra Shah, *Everything You Should Know About Chelation Therapy* (Atlanta: '76 Press, 1997), 18.
3. Elmer M. Cranton, M.D., *Bypassing Bypass* (Charlottesville, VA: Hampton Roads Publishing, 1990), 33.
4. Ibid.
5. Ibid., 34.
6. Walker, *Everything You Should Know About Chelation Therapy,* 16.
7. Cranton, *Bypassing Bypass,* 18.
8. Source obtained from the Internet: www.americanheart.org.
9. Source obtained from the Internet: Foreword to *A Textbook on EDTA Chelation Therapy,* ed. Elmer M. Cranton, M.D., www.drcranton.com/chelation/linus_pauling.htm.
10. Ibid.
11. Source obtained from the Internet: http://drcranton.com/newhope.htm#WHAT%20TYPES%20OF%20EXAMINATIONS.
12. Ibid.
13. Ibid.
14. Ibid.

CHAPTER 14:
THE BEAT GOES ON

1. Sherwin Nuland, *The Mysteries Within* (New York: Simon & Schuster, 2000), 184.
2. Source obtained from the Internet: www.magnet.mt/health/impaedcard/issue/issue1/csv/csv.htm#top.
3. Karl Taube, *Aztec and Maya Myths* (Austin: University of Texas Press, 1993).
4. Nuland, *The Mysteries Within,* 185.
5. Robert Erickson, *The Language of the Heart: 1650–1750* (Philadelphia: University of Pennsylvania Press, 1997), 26.
6. Ibid., 3.

7. Ibid., 1–2.
8. Nuland, *The Mysteries Within,* 16.
9. Ibid., 186–187.
10. See note 2.
11. Erickson, *The Language of the Heart,* 3.
12. Moore, *Heart Failure,* 18.
13. Erickson, *The Language of the Heart,* 4.
14. Nuland, *The Mysteries Within,* 199.
15. Erickson, *The Language of the Heart,* 4.
16. Ibid., 12.
17. Ibid., 2.
18. Source obtained from the Internet: *The Columbia Encyclopedia,* 6th ed., www.bartleby.com/ 65/ri/Richard1.html.
19. Source obtained from the Internet: www.concordance.com/ cgi-bin/1wrdr.pl.
20. Erickson, *The Language of the Heart,* 16.
21. Ibid., 12.
22. Source obtained from the Internet: University of Toronto, http://dante.med.utoronto.ca/skeletalmuscle/history.htm.
23. See note 19.
24. Phillip E. Johnson, *Defeating Darwinism* (Westmont, IL: InterVarsity Press, 1997), 10.

CHAPTER 15

TAKE HEART

1. Source obtained from the Internet: The Franklin Institute Online, www.fi.edu.
2. Sian Griffiths, *Predictions: 30 Great Minds on the Future* (Oxford University Press, 1999).
3. Ibid.
4. Susan A. Greenfield, *Journey to the Centers of the Mind* (W. H. Freeman & Co., 1995).
5. Simopoulos, *The Omega Diet,* 96.
6. Source obtained from the Internet: Sean McMann, "Angry response to everyday life can cause health problems" (June 17, 1996): www.cnn.com/HEALTH/9606/17/ men.and.anger/index.html.
7. Source obtained from the Internet: www.healthwellexchange.com/nutritionsciencenews/ NSN_backs/Sep_98/sinatra.cfm.
8. Source obtained from the Internet: BBC News, "Cash link to gum disease" (July 20, 1999): news.bbc.co.uk/hi/english/ health/newsid_398000/398474.stm.
9. Source obtained from the Internet: Brooke C. Wheeler, "Can You Die of a Broken Heart?" www.allhealth.com/health/followup/print/0%2C4197%2C6723 _173148%2C00.html.

10. Source obtained from the Internet: Denise Mann, "Depressed? You May Be More Likely to Develop Heart Disease: Study Finds a Strong Connection; It's Not Clear Whether Treatment Helps," WebMD Medical News (October 10, 2000): my.webmd.com.

11. Marilyn Elias, "Exercising my fight depression in the long run," *USA Today* (January 11, 2001): 1D.

12. Source obtained from the Internet: Amy Norton, "Unhappy marriages may harm women's hearts" (March 13, 2001): Reuters Ltd., Center for Cardiovascular Education, www.heartinfo.org.

13. Bill Thomsom, "The Second Act of Dean Ornish," *Natural Health* (November/December 1998).

Suggested Reading

Brecher, Harold and Arline. *40-Something Forever* New York: Health Savers Press, 1992.

Cassileth, Barrie R., Ph.D. *The Alternative Medicine Handbook.* New York: W.W. Norton & Company, 1998.

Cranton, Elmer. *Bypassing Bypass.* Troutdale, VA: Hampton Roads, 1990.

Halstead, Bruce. *The Scientific Basis of EDTA Chelation Therapy.* Colton, CA: Golden Quill Publishers, Inc., 1979.

Heimlich, J. *What Your Doctor Won't Tell You.* New York: Harper Collins Publishers, 1990.

Trowbridge, John. P., and Morten Walker. *The Healing Powers of Chelation.* Stamford, CT: New Way of Life, Inc., 1992.

Index

Receive
3 Issues of
Charisma
& CHRISTIAN LIFE
FREE

Compliments of
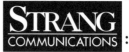

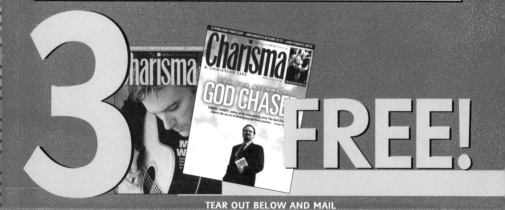

TEAR OUT BELOW AND MAIL

CHARISMA magazine
* the Country's Leading Christian Publication!

FREE Offer Certificate

☑ **YES**, I'd like to receive a FREE 3 MONTH (3 issues) subscription to **CHARISMA** magazine. I understand that I am not obligated to make any additional purchases and that this is a FREE offer.

Name _____

Address _____

City_____ State_____ Zip _____

Telephone_____

E-mail _____

Valid in the USA only.   9IGHRT

*based on newstand sales

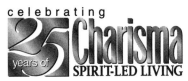

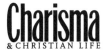